DADDY

Tish Granville and Lanelle Jackson

DADDY HUNGER

Feeding the Deficit With Divine Dining

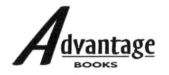

Tish Granville
and
Lanelle Jackson

Library of Congress Catalog Number: 2022933429

First Printing: June 2022
22 23 24 25 26 27   10 9 8 7 6 5 4 3

Table of Contents

INTRODUCTION

Missing Dads
Another Type of World Hunger

Everyone knows what hunger is or what it feels like to be hungry, but there are some people who know the feeling all too well. The United Nations Food and Agriculture Organization (FAO) estimates that 820 million people are suffering from hunger throughout many parts of the world daily.[1] Many of us who are considered well off in life can go a few hours without a meal before proclaiming—and falsely—that we are starving. The truth is many of us don't know the half of what starvation really is.

Starvation, which often leads to malnutrition and even death, is a way of life for many across the world. Some of us experience hunger because we simply forgot to eat or were too busy to eat while others with real hunger problems live in a constant state of scarcity, meaning they don't have the resources to get food regularly.

The issue of hunger is all around us. It's in our backyard and stretches far across the oceans into foreign lands. It's in our school systems, homes, and communities. It's in every city, state, country, and continent. We have all witnessed scenes of individuals on street corners begging for spare change and food, to scenes of homeless individuals digging through random trash receptacles. We've observed commercials of organizations imploring people to help starving children in various countries and we've participated in fund-raisers and missions set in place to help children around the world eat at least one meal every day.

We cannot deny that hunger is a real and observable problem around the world and in our own country. Hunger is described as an uneasy sensation occasioned by the lack of food.[2] It is also a strong desire or craving. World hunger is described as the want or scarcity of food in a country and across the world.

We can clearly see that world hunger is a major problem worthy of attention and action, but we want to draw your attention to an equally devastating problem, that in our opinion needs intense awareness and action. We are talking about Daddy Hunger here, and that daddy hunger is due to the alarming rate of missing fathers in homes in the US. The missing father epidemic, and yes, it is an epidemic, has been plaguing homes in America for many years and it is seemingly getting worse.

According to The National Fatherhood Initiative, there are 18.3 million children in America who live in fatherless homes.[3] That is an alarming "one-out-of-every-four" children. It is unsettling to imagine that as many children are in fatherless homes, there is a plethora of children-less fathers. Yes, for every fatherless child, there is some father roaming around and living his life without his child or children by his side. This is saddening and even frustrating.

We wish we could interview all the dads in the world and find out what their reasons are for not being in their child's life. We can only suspect they are uninvolved due to poor self-esteem, lack of finances, lack of skill, fear, being kept away by the mother, being incarcerated, unawareness of offspring, being busy with work and travel, feeling unprepared, and the list goes on. We are certain that many share the sentiment that there are not enough reasons in the world to not be involved in your child's life. Regardless of a father's hang-ups, his absence can lead to a long list of unnerving issues.

Here are some of the negative impacts that an absent father can have on children:

- Children in fatherless homes are at 4 times greater risk of poverty.

- Infant mortality rate in fatherless homes is higher than married-couple homes.

- Children with involved fathers in the home have higher academic achievement and success.

- Children with single mothers tend to have higher levels of aggression and problematic behaviors.

- Adolescent girls from fatherless homes are 7 times more likely to become pregnant.

- Children raised in fatherless homes are at risk for abusing drugs later and they are more likely to commit crimes.

These are just a few statistics that The National Fatherhood Initiative derived from the U.S. Census Bureau 2020 report.[4] These do not fully entail many of the unreported and real-life issues that fatherless children and adults endure. We wish we didn't have to explain the importance of the presence of a father, but we must assume there are many uninformed individuals in the world who do not truly know the purpose of a father. A simple look at the daily news, a walk through a local school, visiting a child at their home, visiting a detention center, and going to the city jail are proof that the inexistence of fathers in the home is both detrimental and destructive to the individuals, the homes, and the community at large.

Fathers are meant to be the pillars of the homes. They are there to provide protection, structure, harmony, stability, support, love, and financial resources. They are not just, or at least they should not just be there to take up space. They are vital to every mother's ability to help run the home and certainly to bring an emotional balance to the child or children in the home. It has become all too common and even oddly normal to not have a father in the home.

Individuals who grow up without a father are at serious risk for facing a wide range of psychological, relational, emotional, spiritual, economical, and behavioral issues. This includes mental health problems, instability in life, low self-esteem, poor relationships with others, poor money management, difficulty making decisions, or anger issues. And trust us, this is a small list of the possibilities of what a fatherless individual could face in life. We know this because we have lived it. We have lived with our own concoction of emotional, spiritual, and psycho-social issues.

That is why writing this book was so important to us. Not only do we want to share our story of growing up without a father, but we want to reiterate the importance of a father, the devastating effects of him being missing, and offer hope that not even a missing father should keep someone in bondage for their entire life.

There is so much hope in God as our Abba father and He is so mighty that He can take the broken pieces of someone's life and instill the best parenting that anyone could ever receive. No, we do not want to minimize the role of an earthly father. They are put here for a purpose and to represent Christ in the homes. However, we do want to maximize the role of God the father.

As you journey through the pages of this book, you will observe the realness and pain of growing up fatherless, but you will also observe the sovereignty of God and how He has always been there to fill the paternal void.

CHAPTER 1

WHAT IS DADDY HUNGER?

*"The hunger for love is much more difficult to remove
than the hunger for bread."—Mother Teresa*

When a person is hungry, it is a physiological signal; an innate desire
or need for food. It is one of those undeniable indicators that a need must
be fulfilled. You can't ignore it.... well you can, but ignoring hunger
makes you no less hungry. We were created to need food to survive and
thrive. You can only survive so many days without food before
deterioration and ultimately death becomes your fate. Hunger for food is
inherent. It is built within you and there is nothing you can do about it,
except honor this hardwired natural instinct and eat something.

This book is about another type of hunger. Daddy hunger. This is the
hunger we had to endure from birth until now. While we truly want to be
sensitive to our primary caretakers, the culture in which we were raised,
the circumstances surrounding our conception, and the life stories of those
before us, we also want to honor our own story, our own culture, our own
voices, and our understanding of God's plan for families. And His design
was for children to have their fathers in their lives. He set it up that way
and any deviation from His blueprint causes pain, no matter the
circumstances that caused the deviation to occur.

We don't blame, shame, or name in this book. When something goes
wrong in life, it is human nature to want to find someone or something to
blame. The culture we live in is very much an *at-fault* culture. While we
believe in truth-telling, justice, and accountability, we have learned the
power of forgiveness, radical acceptance, and mercy and want that to be
the tone of this book. If for some reason, a different tone is expressed,
please accept that as our personal lamentation and our need to accurately

name our grief. God allowed this to be our painful story and now we want to share it with the world—that we are here today, scars and all, to showcase God's faithfulness, goodness, and love that lifted us out of the pain of fatherlessness.

We also want to be sensitive to those who have daddy hunger due to other circumstances such as death or other life variables that caused dad to be unavailable—like military service, very demanding careers, or life-long and incapacitating illnesses. We understand that there are many versions of father wounds, but this book is primarily about daddy hunger due to a father not being present in the home. This is our rendering of what it feels like to grow up without a father and endure daddy hunger.

So, what is daddy hunger? Daddy hunger, in our definition, is having a desire, craving, or need for a dad. If physical hunger is the result of a lack of food, then daddy hunger is the result of a lack of a father. Sometimes hunger manifests due to scarcity of food—sometimes there is food and sometimes there isn't, or maybe it's available in insufficient quantities. Our daddy hunger isn't because of scarcity of a father, it's due to 100% absence—we have never met our father or had the experience of knowing a father. It is worth noting that since 2020, we have teamed up with a high school friend that is gifted in genealogy, family trees, and searching for bio-parents and we are on a more intentional and hopeful path to discovering our biological father and paternal family.

Daddy hunger is a need for daddy

Growing up without a primary attachment figure is an incredible grief experience. Many may wonder how you can grieve something you never really had—because we never had a father to lose. But to the contrary, not ever meeting our father is a great loss because his seed is responsible for our even being here. We had him to pro-create us; we lost him after that. So, it is a loss to grieve.

Children need their fathers. A need suggests something that is a requirement, something that is necessary. When needs are unmet, conditions tend to be difficult or maladaptive. Well-being is compromised in the absence of what is needed in life. Survival tends to be jeopardized.

Thrive-ability is at stake. Endangerment is likely when certain needs are consistently lacking.

Having a hunger for daddy in the form of a need for us indicated that our dad was required and necessary in our lives. Because he was absent, the condition of our lives was undoubtedly difficult and at times negative. Our wellbeing or ability to "be well" emotionally, spiritually, socially/relationally, physically, and environmentally was compromised through different developmental stages growing up, which we will disclose throughout the book. Obviously, we survived, but that survival was indeed threatened.

Fatherlessness did not necessarily threaten our lives physically, but rather threatened our lives in every other way. When you go through life without a significant need being met, you must learn how to survive. To survive is to remain alive or continue to exist despite some unfortunate occurrence. We had to play the hand we were dealt. Sometimes survival means doing the best you can with what you have. It means taking it one day at a time because the very thought about tomorrow is just plain scary.

Lacking something vital such as a father also jeopardized our thrive-ability. To survive and thrive are different concepts. To thrive is to flourish. It is going above and beyond survival by prospering and being successful despite threats. We needed our dad not only to give us survival tools but to be our survival tool because of what fathers offer their daughters in life. We needed him to thrive—to flourish and go above and beyond day-to-day survival. He was key to us having the tools to bloom and prosper.

Although we live in a liberal society that suggests new definitions of family that can function just fine without a father, according to God's model, fathers are necessary. They are necessary beyond procreating. They are necessary beyond helping to fertilize an egg. They are necessary beyond a wild and passionate night with mom. Fathers are necessary for the growth and development, leadership and love, protection, and provision of every child.

We are so grateful for the seed that got us here because our birth and life on this earth was destined; it is so purposeful and will continue to be meaningful. But we needed so much more than a seed facilitating our in-utero growth. We needed daddy outside of the womb. We needed him to help raise us, lead us, love us, protect us, and provide for us.

Much of our young lives we had very little explanation for why we didn't have a father. It must have been a taboo subject because it was never brought up. Maybe the hope was that we wouldn't notice that we didn't have a father and that if enough days went by, we would adapt to not having such a vital figure in our lives and adapt to the hunger.

Well, the hunger never went away, and we noticed he wasn't around, and we certainly knew something was wrong with the picture. Kids are smart. God made fathers and he put inside of children an innate need for one. There is no amount of silence or lack of conversation or ignoring that can make that innate need go away. Period.

Daddy hunger is a desire for daddy

Not only did our hunger indicate a need for a daddy, but our hunger also signaled a desire for one. Needing something and desiring something are two different experiences. You can desire something without necessarily needing it and need something without necessarily desiring it. A desire is a longing or a want. It is to wish for something that brings satisfaction or enjoyment. We wanted dad. We wanted him around and we had a hard time managing that desire.

Growing up, some well-meaning friends would tell us that we were better off without a father because they didn't get along well with theirs. In a sense what they were saying was that they did not desire their fathers. They didn't find satisfaction or enjoyment in their father-child relationship. They may have needed what their fathers provided, such as financial resources and protection, but they were lacking the warmth and chemistry that connects fathers and daughters. Now that we are older, we understand that having the physical presence of a father does not guarantee desirous emotions. Scripture instructs fathers not to exasperate their children in Ephesians 6:4, and perhaps when exasperation happens, children lose their desire for daddy. But for two little girls who had nothing to work with, we wished for and desired daddy with reckless abandon.

We imagined the satisfaction and enjoyment having a father would bring us. When your reality is less than favorable, that's when imagination takes over for a kid. Our desires for daddy lead us into a fantasy life where we conjured up the joy of having a father by simply imagining having one. That's one thing no one could take away.

Daddy hunger is a craving for daddy

Cravings can be very overwhelming. They can be irrational and illogical. Cravings can come at you like a flood and take you under with one crashing wave. It can be hard to focus when you are craving something, as you become tunnel-focused on the object of your craving until you obtain it. This is often how we responded to the absence of our father. It felt like hunger with a vengeance. Sometimes it was hard to think straight especially when we were exposed to other two-parent families.

Cravings can take over your judgment in certain contexts because oftentimes, cravings are directed towards unhealthy objects—like cupcakes or cigarettes. Cravings can be directed toward things that logically you should not or cannot have or enjoy. But cravings can also be pointed towards healthy things like a salad or a hug.

What Daddy Hunger is Not

Daddy hunger is not a diagnosis that needs to be pathologized. Being hungry for your father does not make you sick or unstable. But it does carry symptoms that need to be cared for, addressed, and attended to. It is not a license to victimhood. As licensed mental health professionals, we have sat with clients who are averse to naming the darkness in their stories, naming perpetrators of harm or giving themselves a label because these confessions or admissions make them to feel like a victim. Confessing that you have a father wound or father hunger does not make you a magnet for pity—it makes you a beneficiary of exhaustive healing. It is not a pass for you to ignore your personal responsibility in life while blaming the consequences of your choices on daddy hunger.

By now, you have a general sense of what daddy hunger is and a bit about what it is not. What feelings and thoughts are coming up for you as you begin to think about hunger in this way? How would you define your relationship with your father using the terms we defined—do you notice needs, desires, or cravings in that relationship? Or maybe you are allowing yourself to have a deeper level of compassion for someone you know who may suffer from daddy hunger? Whatever you noticed, just allow yourself to be curious as we move ahead.

CHAPTER 2

THE DAD-SIZED VOID

"We cannot fill an internal void with an external remedy."
–Graham Elkin

"Death has a finality to it that abandonment simply does not."
–Hope Edelman

The Childhood Years

Jessica was busy in her bedroom playing with her dolls when her playing was halted after hearing the garage door opening. Jessica was only four, but she knew what that sound meant. She ran excitedly to the kitchen, with doll-in-hand of course and waited with expectation for the door to open. Jessica's mother stated calmly "Settle down Jess, move out of the way so your dad can get in the door!" But little Jess was so excited; there was no settling her down. As Jess's mom attempted to scoop her out of the way, the kitchen door flew open and Jess wiggled out of her mother's grasp and ran screaming, "Daddy, daddy!" as she jumped into his arms.

Shayla was having a hard time at her school making friends and feeling happy. Instead, she felt lonely, scared, and was sometimes teased. She was only in the third grade, but certainly felt the pressure of trying to fit in. Leaving school one day in downcast spirits, her father asked her why she looked sad as she got into the car, and she explained to him that she didn't like school. By the time they pulled into their home driveway, she was smiling and practically skipping. So, what happened in the car ride home? Glad you asked—her beloved father spent the entire car ride telling her how beautiful, amazing, important, and brave she was.

These treasured and heartwarming scenes can be imagined so vividly, but unfortunately, they are scenes that many little girls and boys will only imagine. Although these scenes depict the healthy nature of a father-child relationship, they can feel far-fetched and much like a fairytale to a child with a dad-sized void. They, like us, do not have a reality that matches these scenarios.

As we reflect on our formative years, we must express how grateful we are that our young children get to experience life with fathers. Our children will not have to rely on their imaginations to fill in the details of what a father void causes. Although we do not have any experiences of our father scooping us up and spinning us around in the air until we got dizzy or bringing us sweet treats home, we are blessed that our children will have these opportunities.

The early years of our lives entailed a lot of great memories: school, church, road trips, fun holidays, weekend mall trips, tons of playtime, laughter, and fellowship. We cannot say we had a terrible childhood, even with some very troublesome memories. It is possible that our distractions with having so much fun with our toys took our minds away from the big void or that missing person in all the photos.

In our home of origin, certain things were not discussed. We never had the pleasure of receiving much comfort for our loss. We never had any heart-felt talks or attempted explanations as to why our father was missing, at least none that we can remember in detail. The only thing we ever heard was "You guys have a family who loves you and that's all that matters." But to us, there was more, a lot more that mattered to us.

We were small, but we were not blind. When we watched TV sitcoms and saw the popular TV dads, we knew dads existed. We saw kids at school get picked up by their dads from school. Even more, God placed in our precious young hearts a desire for our earthly father. Whether or not our caregivers tried to ignore the issue or keep us distracted from caring, we felt an innate desire for him.

A lot of times parents and family members keep silent about things because they are internally conflicted on if sharing details of what they know will cause more harm than good, and we get that. It's an uncomfortable place for anyone to be in; bringing up difficult topics that are seemingly better off left swept under a rug. Well, if we're talking about sweeping things under a rug, this is more of an elephant being forced under a rug. The silence ended up being emotionally catastrophic for us! Sometimes the most dangerous thing for kids is the silence that allows them to construct their own stories—stories that almost always cast them as alone and unworthy of love and belonging.[1]

One thing about us is that we loved to play pretend with our Barbie dolls and baby dolls. It is quite interesting and possibly even strange to some that we were jealous of the lives that our Barbie dolls had—the make-believe lives that we had given them. Typically, children act out or play out the actual events that they experience based on what we have observed in actual therapy sessions as professional clinical counselors and in research. That is why we, along with other mental health therapists rely on play therapy techniques to see what is going on in the minds of young children. However, we did not play out what we lived. No—we played out what we desired. Our Barbie dolls were not portrayed as single mothers nor were they living in a home full of extended relatives. Our Barbie dolls were happily married with 1-2 children, a dog, and a beautiful home. No fighting, no chaos, no drama, no brokenness in our Barbie worlds.

Therefore, we were jealous. We imagined all this pretend play, but we also became so involved that we really felt Barbie had something we did not have—the family we truly wanted.

The same was true for our pretend 'house' or baby doll play. We envisioned ourselves as loving wives with several children and it always felt so comforting to imagine what we wanted.

Why did we spend so much time pretending some might ask? One reason is pretending and spending so much time playing provided us with a great escape. The more we played—the less gloomy our reality looked. Some of our family members can attest to the number of hours we would spend out on the back porch or in the basement just blocking out the world. We only took breaks to eat or use the bathroom. Pretending fully took our minds off certain pains. Sunup to sundown we were in a pretend world.

We recall waking up at sunrise and running straight to our Barbie stash to begin constructing our make-shift interpretation of a dream home and immediately getting lost in a world that was so different from our own. If we did have to stop playing, we rushed through whatever we had to do to get back to playing again. It was serious! And if our caretakers ever called us for something, we became so agitated that our play was being interrupted. The same was true for the phone ringing or, even worse, nighttime approaching. Once it started getting dark, we started wrapping up our scripts so we could end our play in an organized fashion. It was almost like a soap opera the way we organized our Barbie play. We hated—absolutely hated to stop!

Why are we detailing all of this? Simple—some very fortunate kids' worlds involved playing outside with their dads or even both parents and spending time with them daily. Since we didn't have that, over-indulged fantasy Barbie play was our next best thing.

The second reason we pretended so much is that we were displaying faith without even realizing what we were doing. If faith is seeing what is not there before actually seeing it, then we did this every time we played. As young kids, we may have been presumptuous to believe our father would one day appear and change our lives forever, but we believed it and we also believed that when we got older, we would have our own complete families. We played out what we one day wanted to have. We were laser focused. We only pretended to have a family with a husband, wife, and children. Never anything else. Our present state at that time was not enough to deter what we wanted. To us, a home just was not right without a father.

Along with the excessive pretend play, we also had countless moments of wishing on shooting stars, making birthday wishes, and using wishing wells to bring our dad to us one day. Just imagine being a little girl watching a shooting star fly across the night sky and praying fervently and deeply to God that He would grant a special wish. We heard so many nursery rhymes and fairy tale songs on wishing on a star, and we believed wishes could come true that way. We dumped out coin purses into wishing wells and even those plastic wishing wells displayed at grocery stores hoping at least one of those wishes would be granted. Other kids would probably want to spend their coins on candy or toys, but not us. We would spend all the money in the world to know our father. Birthday after birthday, year after year, we closed our eyes wishing to meet our father one day. No one ever knew what we were wishing for, but we did. We never gave up hope that one day one of our many wishes would come true.

The Teenage Years

Growing up without a father in the childhood years was certainly hard, but not quite as hard as the teenage years. During the childhood years, children are somewhat aware and very impressionable. In the teenage years, individuals are very aware and three times more impressionable. Teenagers tend to investigate things more on their own and ask more questions, not so much out of innocent curiosity like children, but out of intentional and goal-directed curiosity. They want to know not just why, but who, when, what, where, and how.

In the teenage years, the unanswered questions or the lack of information given led us to believe that no one cared or that the people around us were intentionally trying to hurt us. We felt as if everything else was more important than helping us understand why we did not have a father. In our minds, the silence or the lack of empathy and concern shown was just the same as shoeing us away and saying, "get over it." It just did not seem right or fair that we were left to suffer silently.

It is hard enough being a teenager with major self-image issues, low self-esteem, and trouble fitting in. On top of that to have "daddy" issues is simply overwhelming. This was our plight as teenagers. We struggled to fit in. Not so much as far as making and keeping friends. We were able to be sociable and adapt to whatever social group or network we chose to. It was more feeling insecure about how we came across to people or how we looked compared to everyone else. We wanted people to like us, and we wanted to seem cool and hip without compromising our standards, but it was hard at times. We did not really have the hip clothes, hair, or get to do things other kids got to do.

So not always looking the part and not having the same privileges as most kids oftentimes impacted the way we felt about ourselves. We felt bad about ourselves as teens, and sadly, we did not have the love and care of an earthly father to come in and remedy our low self-esteem with hugs and positive affirmation. While it is true that a lot of dads do not necessarily do adequate jobs of building up their kids, we would like to focus on the dads that do and how we needed that support during that time.

We can just imagine how drastically different things may have been for us had we been blessed with the kind words of a father maybe after a bad day at school or maybe he would catch us in the mirror beating ourselves up and he would press his head against ours and say, "I think you look beautiful!" We can only imagine how much better we would have felt being thrown in a vicious world of competition, pressure, and drama called teenage years. We wonder what advice or wisdom he might have given us about homework, friendship, boys, heartache, being safe, God, our futures, or our dreams. To be honest, we do not even know what kind of dad he would have been in general or if he would have been partly there, a rolling stone, spiritually lost, street, very involved, righteous, strict, or humorous. All we know is we needed someone back then and, in some ways, we still need him now.

It was not uncommon at all to see other teens and friends of ours without fathers in their homes either. It was a plague of missing fathers and we saw the effects it had on other friends as well, but it still felt like we were on island all by ourselves. When it came to not having a complete family, it seemed like we were the only ones suffering. Suffering how? In many ways: emotionally, spiritually, physically, and relationally. We will look at the specific ways that we suffered later in book. We are just thankful that we did not become troubled youth and get into bad situations. We had many issues, but God certainly shielded us from making a lot of negative life-changing choices.

The Adulthood Years

Not having a father at any stage of life can certainly be challenging, but the pain and challenges that are presented during adulthood seem more intense. We do not know exactly what makes the pain more intense, but it could possibly be attributed to the fact that adults are a lot more aware, and the brain is fully developed to feel, think, and respond. Also, the 20–30-year-old span of development is often characterized by formation of identity, figuring out life, organizing relationships, spiritual development, and deeper self-reflection. Honestly, the 20-30's period is often when adults realize just how wounded they really are.

Once we became adults and went off to college, we knew we had a huge void, and we also knew exactly what to do to try and cope with it. We talked more with each other about our feelings and discussed our disappointments. We felt an urgency to be the best that we could be and keep pressing through life, but while we pressed through life, the pain of not having a father pressed on us. We could not escape how broken we often felt and at times, still feel.

As young adults we did not let go of our coping skills used in childhood. We still found ourselves daydreaming a lot, wishing on stars, and using writing and art to express our true longing. We started writing a lot actually! We wrote poems, journal entries, and fake letters. It is hard to stop doing these things because we yet believe that these methods help us heal to some degree.

There were periods of times though where we really were not aware of our void and just lived our lives. We had so much fun in college and striving for our goals that a missing father just was not at the top our priorities—or so we thought. I, Lanelle can recall a particular event during my freshman year of college where I needed some test-taking help from the school psychologist and it lead to a huge 'aha' moment for myself and later my sister. During my first session, the clinician did a very normal and standard interview asking me about my upbringing and where my mother and father were.

Once I disclosed the absence of a father, it opened a huge door that I was not ready for. I was just concerned about getting over my test anxiety when she was more concerned that I had 'daddy issues.' "Daddy issues? Me? No way Doc! I'm on my way to a bonfire with friends; I don't want to hear this!" But she was right. I immediately went back to the dorm in tears and shared with Tish and we both cried.

It was an awakening of sorts. Yes, we had missed our father throughout childhood and teenage years, but somehow, we began to ignore the issue during college, and it came back and hit us both like a bus. We were shocked and emotional for days. We were confronted with feeling a new wave of pain because it felt different as an adult to acknowledge pain.

It took—it takes more intentional responsibility to look at pain as an adult. It is more profound—more defined.

So, there we were with the all-so-familiar question "Where is our father?" And still no answers. The clinician shifted our focus completely and challenged us to find answers and it was then that we began a journey to find those answers. We came up with a plan to write our mother a letter and asked to have an open discussion. We did eventually have a conversation and while we will not disclose the details of the conversation, the end result was pretty much a dead-end. While we had no definite answers at that time, possibly 20 years ago, we now know more information and we are hopeful that our research and searching will soon pay off.

CHAPTER 3

THE HUNGER PANGS

"My tears have been my food day and night"- Psalm 42:3

Just when you try to emotionally and intellectually disconnect from the very thing that you need, the body screams at you, "I'm hungry!" There is no denying with your head what the body is experiencing when you are hungry for food. Your body will turn on you. And anyone who's ever been hungry before knows this.

Everyone has had an angry bear in his or her stomach before, or in other words had their stomach growl. It's that not-so-subtle rumbling noise the stomach makes when it is time for food. Stomach grumbles don't care if you are in class, church, asleep in your bed, spending time with a friend or loved one, or in a meeting when it interrupts. It often is embarrassing and dreadful. If this growling happens in the earshot of others, you can guarantee someone will remind you that its time to eat.

But hunger is about more than the sound, it is about the feeling. Hunger pangs are contractions that happen when the walls of the stomach begin to rub against each other around 12-24 hours after the last meal. This is a very uncomfortable feeling that is also referred to as hunger "pangs"—a sign that it is time to eat.

This is all a mechanism of the inherent wisdom in our bodies that is set to help us survive by not allowing us to starve. The discomfort is purposeful. Well, the same is true about our experience growing up without a father. It was a lot of growling and a lot of pangs. Our childhood, adolescence and young adulthood was full of contractions and noise to remind us that we were hungry for daddy.

Just like hunger pangs for food are hard to ignore, it was hard all these years to ignore what we were sensing and experiencing with no one to call "dad."

OWNING THE PANGS

There is so much about life in general that enables the presence of pain in each one of our lives. If you have never experienced anything painful, we don't know that you are truly human. If you have never had anything happen to you that scarred you, caused you to shed a tear, lose your breath, ask God "why?", or hurt your feelings, you might want to check your pulse. If you are human, you should have at least one painful experience in your historical timeline.

While we have many different negative life events we can attest to, growing up without a father is by far the most painful one. Pain is a very subjective emotional experience. This simply means that what is painful for one person may not be painful at all for another person. Pain is personally defined. Everyone deserves the right to judge his or her own experiences as either painful or pleasant. Pain cannot be compared from one person to the next nor should we judge another person's pain. Therefore, we have a problem with the use (or should we say the misuse) of words like "weak" and "strong."

Typically, when you do not handle loss well, when you cry from time to time, when you share your distress with others with a solemn disposition, when you grieve or have a hard time bouncing back, people will label you as "weak." To earn a label of "strong" or have someone praise your courageous attitude toward a loss, you must smile a lot, jump back on the fast-moving train after a hurt, display a false sense of joy and peace, and suppress your tears.

What a tremendous amount of pressure! With that in mind, it is well understood that there are thousands of other women (and men) who grew up without a father who would agree that their predicament was painful for them, while there are countless others who would rate it as a minor setback. "To each his own" as they say. This is where we allow one another to experience fatherlessness differently and uniquely.

It's ok to own your own pain if there is a relationship you have suffered hunger from. To own your own pain/pangs just means to be courageous enough to admit you are in pain and to avoid waiting for others to tell you that you have pain that you need to deal with. For some people, owning the pain may mean turning it into something sacred. For others it may mean disclosing the pain to those you love, to say, "Hey you know a lot about me, but what you don't know is I have this pain or this hunger I've been keeping suppressed." For others, acknowledging that you are in pain is the genesis of healing—because if we cannot admit we have hunger pangs, we cannot effectively heal. Not being able to acknowledge by words how you feel or connect with your pain is referred to as alexithymia.[1] Overcoming the barrier of not being able to share your pain is key to overcoming the pain! Sometimes pain submerges until it can find a pathway for expression or resolution.[2]

Owning does not mean using your pain as a crutch or using your hunger for secondary gains and to manipulate those around you. Owning does not mean staying stuck. It does not mean clamoring for pity. If you are interpreting or demonstrating ownership in that way, you can change your perspective and should consider starting a path toward healing.

In the world of behavioral therapy there is a widely used tool called the "Subjective Units of Distress Scale", developed by a South African psychiatrist named Joseph Wolpe. It is very effective in helping people rate their level of subjective distress, pain, or emotional disturbance. The scale measures distress 0-10 where 0 represents a very neutral experience and 10 represents the worst of whatever the unpleasant emotion is. For the sake of our experience, we will reinvent the scale and call it the Father Hunger Scale. We would rate growing up without a father overall somewhere between a 7-10 in terms of hunger, but different stages of life warranted different ratings. There were times where the pain wouldn't budge from a 10 and then there were other moments, days, or seasons where the pain or hunger was minimal; like a 1 or 2. No matter where we were on the scale, we had to own the pangs. And so do you.

And for the record, just because we are identical twins did not mean that we experienced the same pain. We didn't. Remember, pain is subjective. Each person gets to define where he or she is in relation to pain.

But because we are twins, we did have the opportunity to share a lot of our experience and we did indeed have a lot of overlap in how we felt, how intensely we felt the pain, and how long we endured the pain. But there were plenty of times when one of us was having a hard time and the other could not relate at that moment. We both had our own life experiences and were triggered differently. How we own our pain differs even though we are both hungry from the same father.

If you have not owned your father pain yet, maybe this is a good place to pause and take ownership. If you have been hungry for a father, hungry for love, and enduring the various pangs of missing dad—it's time for you to say, "I admit I have father pain! I'm hungry, I'm hurting, and I want help!"

DADDY HUNGER TRIGGERS

When a person is hungry and they see food, the sight of the food will stimulate activity in the mouth and stomach—salivation and grumbling. They will be reminded of the pain of hunger even if they had temporarily forgotten about it. When you are hungry and don't have access to food in the immediate future, the last thing you want to see is a Chipotle commercial. It might just make you angry. The commercial acts as a trigger.

Pain almost always comes with triggers. Triggers are simply reminders of a painful or traumatic experience one has endured. Triggers are reminders of our true internal condition, meaning we can seem well on the outside until our pain is poked! Triggers activate us within in some way. They stir up our sensations and often remind us of our needs or the lack thereof. These reminders can be little fragments of the pain that aren't painful necessarily on their own, but they represent the fullness of the pain, therefore causing painful reactions apart from the painful event. Another fact about triggers is they cause similar emotional reactions to how one initially responded to the actual painful event, even though the event is no longer happening.

This is because painful events stay lurking around in our brains in the basement of our emotion department. Painful experiences live there until they are stirred up and brought back upstairs to the main floor, or as many refer to as the surface. Pain has a way of seeming like its resolved and hiding in our subconscious mind but rears its ugly head when activated by these things called triggers.

Remember, triggers are mostly benign (harmless). They really don't have power, but they remind us of the event that did have power. Triggers come into our awareness through our five senses: sight, sound, touch, taste, and smell. Our five senses connect us to our pain. They link us back to where it really hurt the worst, whatever "it" is. You can be minding your business, having an awesome day and smell smoke in the air and it can remind you of your neighbor's home that caught on fire when you were five. And you can re-experience the fear and anxiety you had back then as if it were happening now. You can be in a healthy romantic relationship with the love of your life, and they can say something hurtful to you that reminds you of the verbal abuse from your father, which causes you to act out, not because what your mate said was abusive, but because it reminded you of the abuse you endured. These are triggers that activated pain through the senses of smell and hearing.

Now that you understand triggers a little bit better, you will be able to understand how the hunger pangs from not knowing our father were activated by all kinds of triggers in our lives. So many times, we thought we were "over it", healed, thriving through not having a father—and out of nowhere that dormant pain would come alive again because of everyday reminders.

Some of our triggers:

- Seeing two-parent families
- Seeing fathers with their kids
- Movies with happy endings/happy two-parent families
- Men
- Men in power
- Boys
- Babies
- Hearing friends talk about their dads

- The word "father"

- Our birth certificates

- Filling out paperwork/medical visits where father's name or father's information is requested

- Father's Day

As you can see, the above are essentially benign or harmless. But they remind us of our pain. Often, they catch us by surprise and other times we can predict that we will be triggered. As you consider your own hunger pangs, what are your triggers or reminders?

THE INEFFECTIVE CRISIS RESPONSE

In the event of crises, whether natural disasters, fires, mass shootings, terrorism, epidemics, or other tragic situations, there is a certain and almost expected level of response to remedy the crisis. Crisis response teams are trained and specialize in bringing aid, support, and relief to those in need. The main objectives of a crisis response unit or volunteer are to ensure stabilization for those who endure such events.

This is not an easy task, but early intervention in times of crisis helps to also mitigate the escalation of distress or the worsening of the victim's condition in the aftermath of the critical incident. If the response is late or ineffective, victims can struggle to return to pre-crisis level of functioning, mind, body, and spirit. When help does not come on time for victims, they can become wary, skeptical, frantic, and distrustful of those in helper roles.

As it relates to the pain we felt in our lives, we often felt that we were in a crisis—a hunger crisis, and that few came to our aid to relieve us or at least to provide effective relief. We felt that we were in distress and suffering with no response team! No crisis units! Little mitigation of stress! This led to a distrust of those in helper roles around us.

Ineffective Communication

During crisis responses, those on crisis teams have a responsibility to communicate effectively with the victims of the specific crisis. Communication serves to address any questions the victims may have, gather the victim's account of the event, assess the needs of the victim, and outline a plan of relief with the victims.

One of the most painful parts about not having a father was the silence in our family about it. While we do not know the rationale for the silence or lack of communication, we hope the rationale was rational.

Now that we are both parents, we anticipate as our children get older, we will have to have some hard conversations with them. We know that children don't need to know everything about adult matters or family matters and discretion must be utilized in communicating with children about negative events that happen within the family. But we also have strong stances regarding "family secrets." One faulty family commandment is "whatever happens in this house, stays in this house" and another non-favorite is "take it to the grave."

Here are some reasons why taking vital family information to the grave is harmful:

- The information being concealed until death could be the key to set someone in your family free.

- The receiver/recipient is robbed of their right to choose how they will respond to the truth.

- Secrets and lies are like mold and yeast. They love dark, concealed places with no ventilation so they can fester.

- Secrets are kept using the rationale that it will protect people from harm, when hiding vital information is what does the most harming.

- It leaves people to assume. Assumptions aggravate the wound.

- Lack of truth creates confusion, and we all know confusion does not come from God. It's truth that sets people free.

- Lack of truth creates unhealthy curiosity. When you are suspicious about secrets in your family you start digging around for answers and often come across more erroneous information.

- Protecting sensitive information may be wise regarding young children, but it's unfair to take information to the grave when those young children are now adults.

- The truth about the family tree is disrupted for generations to come. Even Jesus came from an ugly family tree (not His heavenly one, rather His earthly one). Lies, adultery, betrayal, murder, and deception all preceded him in His family tree.

We are sure there is another side to this argument, possibly even some very good rebuttals. There will always be exceptions, but the argument for keeping secrets will never be as strong as the one for sharing them (regarding certain pertinent family issues).

Silence in our family was not golden. The silence about our biological father just left us with more confusion, more questions, more wishful thinking, false hope, and empty dreams. There is nothing golden about confusion and assumptions. Like mentioned before, assumptions create more wounds and pain. Our assumptions about our father aggravated our hunger for him.

- Does he know about us, and did he abandon us? –Assumption that leads to rejection

- Is he an amazing person who just doesn't know about us? —Assumption that leads to fantasizing

- Is he a bad person who could hurt us? —Assumption that leads to fear

Silence is not golden for another reason. Not having a father was the elephant in every room of our childhood homes. Even a baby elephant of about 200 lbs. and 3 feet cannot be ignored in a room and fatherlessness was an adult elephant. A big, robust, smelly, loud beast that we had to pretend we didn't see, smell, or hear. "Just walk around it, squeeze by it, cover your nose and ears and go play with your toys" seemed to be the message we received.

We woke up day after day and the elephant was still there sitting on our couch—and no one ever told us why that elephant was there. That's how we'd describe the pain of the silence. Maybe just maybe if we had been told early on about the elephant, we could have started grieving from a more appropriate place and could have put our unhealthy assumptions to rest and not lived a life aggravating our wounds. Just maybe.

Insufficient Resources

When trying to recover from a crisis, resources are needed. Resources help connect the survivor back to normalcy and safety. Resources are services, people, places, and things that meet the material and psychological needs of those in recovery. Resources help survivors of crises "get back to living" and even thriving again. In many events of critical stress, you will hear the word resources used a lot. Let's look at some quick examples. For house fire victims, common resources needed are clothes, furniture, housing/shelter, hygiene products, and food. For a sexual assault victim, resources needed may include legal aide, psychological care, support groups, and medical professionals. A person who had a minor bicycle accident will need resources like a first aide kit, maybe a medical professional and maybe a bike repair shop. If the person is homeless and hungry, then food and shelter are without a doubt the resources needed.

The resources required vary depending on the situation and the individual's needs. But the point that is most important to underscore is that there are many severe consequences because of attempting to overcome critical stress without sufficient resources. The longer a person must wait for critical needs to be met, the greater the chances of developing feelings of helplessness and hopelessness; a loss of will to self-help and a loss of hope in the support of others. Sometimes desperation sets in when a person must do things they never thought they would have to do to survive. Sometimes desperation leads to acting outside of integrity or even God's will (i.e., the hungry person who steals food from the grocery store). Yet for others, desperation leads to mobilization and a fight-mode that facilitates finding resources while still managing their integrity.

In fatherless homes and families, there are definite needs that require resourcing. Children who grow up without fathers physically present have a better chance at recovery the more resources are available to them. The appropriate resources help increase the child's recuperation and long-term ability to thrive. Likewise, a decrease in feelings of helplessness and hopelessness overtime is probable with the right people, places, things, and services in place.

We had many resources provided for us growing up that ensured that our hope didn't run dry and our overall ability to help ourselves remained somewhat intact. We had some support that helped address our daddy hunger (to the extent that it could). Yet we can also say there were some key resources not provided or available to us that would have been instrumental in sparing us some chronic distress and unnecessary hunger pangs.

Maybe as a society, we aren't equipped or mobilized enough to both resource and be resourceful for the quantity of fatherless children that exist, but we'd like to see this change, much of which is why we wrote this book. Below are a few ideal resources for this population, specifically fatherless daughters.

Fatherless Daughters Need the Following Resources:

- God
- Connection to a healthy faith community/healthy pastors
- Mentors/coaches
- Free/low-cost community programs
- Journals/diaries
- Extracurricular activities
- Positive role models
- Healthy stepfathers
- Exposure to healthy marriages
- Hobbies
- Libraries/books/education/safe learning environments
- Mental healthcare/Professional Counselors/Lay Counseling
- Safe and adequate housing

Ineffective Disaster Preparedness

After a victim of a crisis survives the conflict, they need proper preparation for the future. They need skill-building and techniques to deal with any residual effects that may arise and any similar crises that they may now be more susceptible to. It is very common for first-time hurricane and flood survivors to be equipped and educated on what to do in the event of another hurricane or flood. A combination of their experience and education helps prepare them for better outcomes in the event of another natural disaster.

We couldn't prepare for the initial predicament of being born fatherless, but we could be educated and equipped for the fallout and all the future relational crises we might face. We were starved of a father, which made us susceptible to a future of hunger pangs. We needed proper preparation to cope with the various famines we could/would encounter throughout our lives—since fatherlessness does come with seasons of crisis, changes in relationships, abandonments, etc. We do not feel we were properly prepared for how to deal with disappointments in future relationships.

But how do you prepare for future famines once you've been starved of a father? What should you stock up on to better survive subsequent relational famines? Let's explore a few necessities.

- Heart Guards-It is very hard to survive bouts of love followed by droughts of love followed by ouches from love. Therefore heart-guards are needed. They protect your heart from unnecessary wounds and unnecessary people who don't mind playing with hearts. We were given guards in our family, but they were the super, ultra, military-grade, extra-defensive kind. We were taught to be over-guarded, distrustful of others, and leery in our encounters with people. If this teaching were scaled back quite a bit, it could have been helpful.

- Self-Love- There will be times people will say they love you, but it won't be shown very well. During these seasons, you need a reservoir of self-love. We were taught how to love God, but we missed out on instruction on how to really love ourselves. This would have helped sustain us during times where we were starved for love from others and missing our dad.

- Self-Regulation- Both a mother and father (or a caring parent figure) are needed to stimulate you when you are shutting down and soothe you when you are panicked as a baby. When disappointments arise in adulthood, you will need plenty of self-regulation skills so that you can spring back to life when going numb and calm down when agitated.[3]

MISSING NUTRIENTS

Fathers have the potential to offer so much to their children to help them develop and grow into healthy individuals, starting from the time they are babies. For instance, dads help with emotional regulation and brain development, while their absence is associated with emotion dysregulation.[4] We will call these many non-tangible relational qualities they provide *Relational Nutrients*.

Relational Nutrients to a child are like food nutrients to the human body. Food nutrients are the elements in food that help sustain the human body and promote life and wellbeing. They ensure that all the parts, organs, and systems in the body continue to work properly. The more nutrients from food that we have, the better we are. The less nutrients we have, the more at risk we are of sickness, disease, and poor bodily functioning.

Relational Nutrients help ensure that children grow and develop emotionally and relationally and have wellbeing in their mind, heart, and spirit, which helps them to be able to thrive socially. A lack of Relational Nutrients leaves children underdeveloped in their social environments, malnourished in relationships, and could lead to heartsickness.

The biological mother and father in an orthodox family setting provide the necessary Relational Nutrients to their child. However, there are many family make-ups that do not fit an orthodox family. So, anyone who is responsible for raising a child will be referred to as a caretaker or attachment figure and assigned the weighty calling of providing the necessary Relational Nutrients.

The types of nutrients provided to each child are often dependent upon specifics about the caretaker like gender, age, maturity level, personality style, personal upbringing, values, and culture/ethnicity. A younger mother in her 20s may provide different nutrients to her child than a 45-year-old mother. A Hispanic may provide different nutrients to his/her child than a Black parent. A person with a rigid personality style will offer different nutrients than a parent with a more flexible personality. A Christian may provide different nutrients to their child than a Buddhist. Following is a look at some typical differences in the Relational Nutrients mothers provide versus those of fathers.

Nutrients That Mothers Offer

Nurture

To nurture something is to promote its growth and development. According to the definition, many would agree that both mothers and fathers promote the growth and development of children equally. However, in practice, women fulfill the role of nurturer to a greater extent than men do. Most men do not qualify themselves as nurturers and many women believe that the lack of a nurturing quality is a weakness. It is almost expected that if you are a woman, you should be nurturing. However, there are many women who do not relate to this quality.

For the sake of this book, we cannot rely on a dictionary definition to expand on our view of this nutrient. We must look at the actual behavior of nurturers to understand why mothers primarily provide this nutrient.

Nurturing to us means tending to the tiniest details in caring for children. It means being hands-on day-in/day-out and meeting the basic needs of children, including feeding, hygienic care, maintaining and restoring health, and taking care of the overall emotional needs of the child. Mothers primarily change diapers, feed/nurse, rock to sleep, get children dressed, take care of children when sick, and just about any other physical need of children. But clearly a robot can do these things. What qualifies these caretaking responsibilities as nutrients versus just actions, is the attitude in which they are done. To be a nutrient these actions must be carried out with warmth, gentleness, attunement, and genuineness.

So, while a mother may just be changing a diaper, there is a chemistry and connection that is transpiring as she does this mundane task, whereas to a non-nurturer, it may be merely a task with no emotional connection.

With daily care being provided with an attitude of warmth, the child grows up feeling loved, noticed, and important. Nurturing lets the child know they are worthy of being cared for as they age, because mom took pride in every need the child had. It's awesome the impact of wiping food off a child's messy mouth.

Affection

Affection ties well with nurture. Affection is a nutrient that is more heavily provided by mothers. Mothers tend to hug and kiss, use terms of endearment, be more excitable in their expressions of love toward their children, use more touch, exaggerated smiles, cuddle, and verbally share their feelings of love and adoration toward their children more than fathers do. For this to be qualified as a nutrient more typical of women does not mean that all women express themselves this way and does not mean that men don't. It simply means most women/mothers find this quality very natural and effortless to express.

Adults who did not have affectionate or nurturing mothers often describe their childhoods and views of their mothers in a more negative tone which says a lot about the importance of this nutrient from mothers. There tends to be a link between lack of affection from mom and intimacy issues later in life. With affection being considered a nutrient, it is supposed to provide children with openness to connection with others, an awareness of safe touch, safe voice/words, and healthy expression of love toward others.

As Christians, we believe love is supposed to consume our children. They shouldn't have to assume if their parents love them or not. No one wants to be in a relationship with someone where they must guess if the person loves them. You won't have to guess if that love is displayed, and often, affection is a means to display love.

Teaching/Learning

To teach means to coach, train, instruct, model, or instill. While fathers are great teachers too of certain lessons, mothers can teach their children a lot about life, manners, daily life activities, independence, and of course God. We strongly believe that parents should be their children's number one educators. Women or mothers tend to take on this role more at times simply because of their availability and constant physical proximity to their children. Dads tend to be busier working from home, caring for other responsibilities or unwinding when at home, so even the best dads still aren't as physically available as moms.

This means that about 75% of what children learn, even without conscious efforts come from mothers. Mothers are constantly teaching their children when to go to sleep, when to wake up, how to be safe and careful in the bathtub, how to say please and thank you, when to be loud or quiet, colors, ABC's, numbers, and the list goes on. Even when moms are quiet, they are still teaching their children using body language.

Mothers being teachers is especially true for the stay-at-home mothers who spend most of their waking hours instilling useful lessons and skills into their offspring. Again, we are not suggesting that dads are not strong teachers as well. In fact, dads need to work alongside moms to instill the teachings of leadership, hope, values, and daily life skills into their children.

Domesticate

When most people think about mothers or domestic tasks, they think of the one who cooks, cleans, does the laundry, and vacuums. Today, while women are still viewed as the ones who primarily engage in these activities, men can and should participate in basic domestic activities. To domesticate simply means to house-train, tame, or discipline—to bring order to. Since the home is filled with so many comforts, those comforts come with responsibilities and the home should be cared for with great effort and responsibility.

That is probably why many mothers spend so much time cooking, and cleaning, and dusting. The responsibility of bringing order to a home requires them to engage in these daily actions. They are doing what is vital to take care of the needs of their families by taking care of the needs of the entire home. Mothers tend to pass on a lot of these responsibilities to children by training them on basic cooking or food preparation skills, doing household chores, and staying organized. This is all a part of domesticating or keeping order. This is a very important role for mothers because many children learn basic life lessons simply by working together to help keep the home in order.

Emotional Intelligence

Research is replete with evidence of the differences in how men and women experience and express emotion. Women are more likely to *befriend* their most vulnerable emotions while men are more likely to *beware* of theirs. Women tend to have more expansive states and ranges, while men tend to be much more restrictive and have limited ranges of emotion. Mothers model this expansive range by talking excitedly on the phone to one of her girlfriends as if she just won a million dollars, showing displeasure or disgust on her face when she finds sticky syrup on the couch from a messy little eater, or screeching with fear when she finds a spider on the wall. Let's be honest, many men do not show such a wide range of emotion. They tend to be more neutral in their facial expressions and non-affective in most situations.

Women tend to take more liberties with their emotions while men often need special authorizations to feel certain feelings. A woman's more liberal style translates naturally into parenting. With her variable expression of emotions, she models a lot about feelings to the children and hopefully how to manage them. Mothers can encourage their children to cry (because they likely see her cry from time to time), let it out, dance around happily, process their feelings, and to process emotions in healthy ways. As an example, we have both implemented feelings charts, calming kits, and toys marketed for helping children build their emotional intelligence with our young children to aid them in their development. Kudos to any dad who has ever bought an emotional intelligence toy for their kid, because that's not the norm.

So, a mother's role to teach emotions is very important. Her ability to allow her own emotions gives space for the child to learn to allow theirs, ideally from a place of wholeness. She should not use her emotions to manipulate, control, or destroy others.

Safety

Safety is strategically placed after the nutrient of emotional intelligence. The more emotionally intelligent mom is, the safer she is. When moms are accepting of all the emotional states of her child, she sends that child the message that they can be human with her. Who wants to be in a relationship where their humanness is condemned? When the world begins to burden the child, they run to mom because her heart is a safe home.

There is an interesting phenomenon that happens between mom and child. When the child is out in the community, he/she finds that they must perform, please, and conform to standards of perfection. When the child returns home to mom, they give up these agendas, which mom often interprets as the child being oppositional and defiant with her. The truth is, he/she knows mom can handle their imperfections and deficiencies. Of course, this does not mean that mom is an emotional punching bag, mom must set boundaries because limits bring safety too.

Structure

Let's just face it! When it comes to structure, mothers tend to be the primary teachers here. Or at least they should be. Mothers are more likely to set bedtimes and organize bedtime rituals, set the dinner time for the entire family, assign homework times, and tell everyone when to go to the bathroom—everyone including her husband if she has one. We are joking, but seriously! The mother's role is so important in keeping everyone on schedule, on time, and on task.

If mom is away or out of town for more than a day, the structure of the home is sometimes at risk for collapse. The home at times turns into a free-for-all. No one eats all day or at least anything healthy. No one brushes his or her teeth. Clothes may be worn inside-out. And homework and school projects may or may not get done. The dog doesn't get walked, the floors don't get vacuumed, and every TV is on in the house. And if the home has smart devices, the children may be in an entirely different part of the house while the father watches from a smart camera. It's as if everyone is excited to have freedom and control for once. But this freedom comes with a price—everyone is hungry, unkempt, and hasn't slept.

God has gifted mothers with the often-overlooked skill of keeping the home structured. Yes, mom may seem unreasonable and overbearing with all her rules, schedules, charts, and limits, but it is her very structure that keeps the home running efficiently. This does not mean that dads are neglectful either. Dads just operate from a different part of their brain that allows for more healthy nonconformity.

Nutrients That Fathers Provide

Affirmation

Affirmation as a nutrient tends to come from fathers. Affirmation is the power of words. Affirmation is building up your child with what you say about who they are, what they do, and where they are going in life. It's more than a nice compliment that goes in one ear and out the other. Affirmations reach down into the deepest parts of a child and tug on their very souls and hearts. Affirmations are more than just your opinion of your child. Affirmations are your truths about your child.

Affirmations from fathers tend to reach a little deeper than affirmation from mothers. Fathers' words tend to have a weightier impact. It is tied to the God-given authority that was placed inside of men.

One scripture that speaks very profoundly about affirmation comes from the Gospel of Matthew 3:17:

And behold, a voice out of the heavens said, "This is My beloved Son, in whom I am well-pleased."

The first thing we observe is that Jesus received an affirmation from the very voice of His Father. It wasn't hearsay. The next thing we notice is that God used a term of endearment—beloved. Thirdly we notice that God the Father showed how He felt proud of His Son. He was "well-pleased" with Him even before his earthly ministry had been recorded to begin. The last and fourth observation is that Jesus received affirmation from His Father before He faced the desert filled with major temptations that He eventually went on to overcome and pass with flying colors.

From these observations in the text, we learn that fathers use their voices to uplift their children. Affirmations are not affirmations unless spoken or even written. A father who thinks kindly about his children is withholding affirmations until he uses his voice to speak to them. Children need to hear praises from their fathers to be well-nourished souls. Fathers also affirm their children by verbally expressing their love for them. Fathers who verbalize that they love their children build strong hearts. Fathers affirm their children by telling them how proud they are of them after they accomplish something. But not just after—before too! Affirmation is a powerful nutrient when dispensed before your child even sets out to complete a task; in other words, a proud father doesn't need the results of their children's actions to celebrate them. Being affirmed before you approach goals really gives you that confidence to be your best. Finally, affirmation helps children face challenges. Jesus received affirmation before He encountered Satan in the desert which ensured that He would persevere through the pressure. Children whose fathers affirm them are better able to withstand peer pressure, life pressure, temptations, crossroads, dark days, and their own personal deserts.

Security/Safety/Protection

We are going to cover these nutrients together because of their strong parallel to each other. Fathers, more so than mothers, are responsible for protecting their children and keeping them safe and secure in the face of threat, danger, harm, and premature death. What a heavy responsibility! Men have more brute strength then women and are built differently in terms of physical capability. Their physical strength is supported with their amazing emotional strength, which knows how to turn off fear and respond to threats with bravery, courage, and confidence.

Men protect in so many ways, from checking the parameters of the house before bedtime, to killing the spider crawling on their little girl's bedroom wall, to jumping in front of the flying baseball headed for their son's head, to much scarier scenarios where their bravery is needed.

A father's fearlessness helps his child to face their own fears or at least feel peace and certainty in the face of fears because of the protection and certainty that dad shows in the face of fears. Many daring children have defeated monsters underneath the bed because dad said, "They can't hurt you because I'm here." And if daddy says it, then it must be true.

When a child feels they can live and thrive without being harmed because of daddy's protection, they develop security. They learn to trust the world they live in and the people who live in it—and when faced with threats or harm they are competent they can survive. Protection is such a vital nutrient to helping children develop security in who they are and in future safe relationships.

To be secure means to be confident and immovable in the face of threat and to be certain of the "good stuff" or the resources you have inside of you no matter what the external circumstances. Fathers help their children to trust the "good stuff" inside and to trust, in a very basic sense, in what is happening around them good or bad. A secure child knows that what is inside of him or her is bigger and better than what is outside. Fathers build this confidence every time they rush to their child's aide, protect, and shield.

Leadership

When God made man, He installed leadership within him. To be a leader is to be in a position of authority and healthy control over a task or a group of people.

Look at the Creation Story when God gave Adam his first chores.

Then God said, "Let Us make man in Our image, according to Our likeness; and let them rule..." Genesis 1:26

The man gave names to all the cattle, and to the birds of the sky, and to every beast of the field. Genesis 2:20

God gave Adam, the first father, permission to rule. He had a busy schedule taking care of all the living creatures and giving them names, making decisions daily about the garden and its upkeep, and providing leadership even though he did not yet have any human followers.

In the same way, fathers have been given leadership over their own "gardens" or homes. Leaders make decisions. Leaders use their best judgment to keep their gardens running smoothly. Leaders don't have to be micromanaged; they have been given the right to rule over designated tasks and they are trusted to do so by God.

A father's primary chore is to run his household, and God has already granted him full permission to do so. A father does not need anyone else to install him into his role. Once a man lies with a woman (hopefully his wife) and conceives with her, he is charged by God to lead that child.

Children need the leadership that fathers provide. They need someone to make decisions that they can rely on. They need someone to have a plan for how "home" will be managed. While the kiddos are tucked in their beds counting sheep at night, they need to trust that daddy is in the next room over pondering how he will lead the family the next day, what decisions to make, which direction to go, which direction to avoid, and reviewing the vision/mission for the family.

Even if daddy must guess sometimes or throw up a hail-Mary, a child wants a father who is comfortable saying "follow me." Most good leaders learned how to lead by watching someone else lead at some point in their life. And oftentimes great leaders came from a home where they had a father providing leadership as a vital nutrient.

Guidance/Direction

This next nutrient may have slight overlap with leadership, but it really stands well on its own. To guide means to provide advice, instruction, and wisdom. If life is one big trip to some predetermined destination, then a map is needed to get to that destination securely. Fathers are often the map, and their job is to help their children get to their destination in life by providing direction. Yes of course mothers can provide much guidance and direction too, but again when we acknowledge the qualities that God instilled within men, we see that he charged men a little differently than He did women.

This may be a bit stereotypical but true nonetheless, but men tend to be a bit more logical (or maybe a lot more logical) than women. They tend to be more spatially oriented and can navigate better than women (literally speaking). There is a scene from a popular movie and book series "Prince Caspian: The Chronicles of Narnia", where the four children are lost trying to find the rest of the Narnians and a very confident Peter questions his younger sister sarcastically, "What? Girls can't carry maps in their heads?" He was implying that guys have a natural gift for exploring the world just fine off instincts.

Apply that to our lives in a figurative sense and you often find that men are very gifted at navigating life very well. Their sense of direction is often quite impressive. When they give life-directions to their children there is a confidence exuded that then gives the child confidence in the path ahead. If daddy said, "go right", then his instruction can be trusted. Children need this so they can stay on course in efforts to reach their individual potential. Without this vital nutrient from dad, children often grow up with a sense of direction-lessness. They often make wrong turns that get in the way of timely arrival to their destination.

Stability

Another key relational nutrient that fathers typically provide is stability. Stability means a pattern of reliability in the environment. Stability often means an absence of unnecessary changes and transitions that disrupt the growth of something. In a sense, it's a basic trust that things will remain consistent.

When a father is dedicated to his family and his children, he tries to create reliability and consistency in the home. He is consistent in taking care of the affairs of the home, he tries to keep his word, he returns home every day, he leads efforts to make sure his family can settle down in one home for a suitable time without interruption, and he has a proven track record of meeting the family's needs.

All these things provide the children with an ability to grow and thrive without anxiety, fear, worry, or confusion. When a child can rely on their home environment to not be up and down like a roller-coaster or round and round like a merry go round, they can settle and thrive without unnecessary interruption.

Without dad in the home to provide this relational nutrient, children are often left feeling vulnerable to change. Now we all know that change is inevitable in life so we are not implying that a father can somehow mitigate the experience of preordained change. But children who grow up in unstable homes because daddy was absent often become change-phobic or change-addicts. Lack of stability makes some people resistant and fearful of change while making others antsy when things stay the same too long. Neither of these extremes are healthy.

Having stability as a relational nutrient fosters a confidence to allow change to happen when it's appropriate and wisdom to not make a habit of inappropriately disrupting your life with too much changing.

Discipline

Discipline as a relational nutrient connects to the God-given authority placed inside of males. Mothers discipline too and do so very well, but the nature of a father's discipline is unparalleled.

We love the scene from The Lion King when Simba runs off for an unapproved adventure to the Elephant's Graveyard. He was already commanded not to go there but he went anyway, and he narrowly escaped a serious threat to his safety. Mufasa was so disappointed in his son that he gave him a firm talking-to. You could see Simba's reverence for his father and embarrassment and fear as he ducked down as if to hide his face from his dad in the field. Mufasa let Simba know his disappointment, the consequences, and his own feelings as a father when his son disobeyed him. Then he used the moment to show his support and protection of his son as they laughed and played in the field.

This portrayed so creatively how fathers have an important job to be firm, protective, and bold in showing their children right versus wrong. Children need this nutrient to have longevity. Discipline prolongs life. Discipline provides boundaries that children need. Discipline is a response to doing things you were told not to do or not doing things that you were told to do. And it's meant to save lives and build character.

I'm sure many people can attest to this scenario: Mom tells her child or children to do something or stop doing something and she gets a partial response or an unsatisfactory outcome. Dad comes home and in one attempt gives the same instruction and gets the desired outcome. It's not because mom is weak, and dad is a bully. It's because mom is more of a nurturer and dad exudes a unique authority.

Children who grow up without a father to provide this nutrient may lack boundaries in their lives that protect them from too many poor choices. They may lack the discipline to execute healthy decisions. They may lack self-discipline: that inner parent that guides them in what to do and what not to do. Discipline also helps children to grow up and recognize limits in their relationships.

It is interesting that we found some very important nutrients that come from a father while we were reading a children's book to our toddlers one day titled "I Love My Daddy Because…." by Laurel Porter-Gaylord. In her book, which is written partly in Spanish, she briefly describes with fun animal illustrations why a child loves their daddy so much. Here are the reasons she lists:

- He plays with me
- He keeps me warm and safe
- He brings me dinner
- He is big and strong
- He takes naps with me
- He can build a house
- He makes me laugh
- He helps me reach things
- He sings me songs
- He takes me for a ride
- He teaches me how to be brave
- He teaches me to be careful
- He plays hide-and-seek with me
- He protects our family
- He watches over me at night[5]

We wish we could unpack some of the roles she highlighted that we did not, but let's investigate a few of them. Dads help their young to reach things. This is both physically and inspirationally. Every small child at some point has been caught in a "too short" situation. You know—too short to reach the sink, too short to reach the toys on the shelf, too short to reach the counter, too short to climb onto the playground set. In many of these situations, kids intentionally call out or run looking for their dads.

It's not that they believe that moms are incapable of helping; it's just engrained in them to depend on a father for these tasks. But dads don't just help their kids reach for things physically. No! They help them reach for their dreams. Reach for great opportunities. Reach for high goals. Dads are essential in helping their children strive for greatness by affirming them and informing them of the potential that lies deep inside of them. So, it's a two-fold role. Dads can help reach the cookies or help their kids try out for a sports team. Whatever he is helping his young to reach, that child has the confidence that they can reach anything if dad has his hand in it.

While some of these vital roles of a father are very fun and seem simple, they all work together to create the total package of a wonderful and fruitful father. We love how she used the illustrations of animals to show that even the birds, beasts, and waterfowl have a useful role for fathers. We believe that God has intended even the highest regard for humans and expects us to parent with the most intentionality, particularly the fathers.

ACCOUNTS OF APPETANCE

Hunger pangs are not fun, especially if you do not have food readily available. The pain of being hungry for daddy was awful because daddy also was not readily available. Many of the significant days and events in our lives had somewhat of an emptiness or incompleteness to them because daddy was not around. These are our accounts of events and experiences we distinctly remember being hungry.

Holidays and Birthdays

Holidays were some of the most memorable times in our family growing up. There are so many blessings growing up with an extended family. When a primary figure is not in your life, having extended family raise and care for you can fill in some gaps and offer a safety net. One of the things our extended family provided for us that we are grateful for is memorable holidays. We honestly cannot remember a "blah" holiday. There was always lots of laughter, family games (that often ended in conflict because of the fierce competition), great & plentiful food, jokes, love, singing, and togetherness.

Christmas had to be our favorite. Every year the Christmas tree would almost be buried underneath all the presents. Everyone in the family received something. No one was left out and being the first grandchildren in the family along with our older sister, we were no doubt spoiled. We had some of the best toys imaginable: Barbie dolls, baby dolls, Legos, tea sets, electronics, board/card games, clothes galore. And since we are '80's babies, we will stretch and say that the '80's produced some of the best toys ever.

After opening awesome presents and then seeing the tree in all its glory standing alone at the end of Christmas day, it left the sound of a blaring silence. Thoughts began to center around the awesome day coming to an end. The fun is over. We've unwrapped our gifts and taken our toys to their designated place in the home. There is no shred of evidence of once wrapped gifts because the garbage has been taken out with all the scraps. There is a stillness in the house that couldn't be heard a few hours ago because of all the joyful noise. And that's when you hear it…. that's when you see it….that's when you feel it! Hear what? See what? Feel what?

Well, that's when you hear the phantom laughter of a father and his daughter while they put together a new toy she received. That's when you see a precious princess sitting on her daddy's lap reading the new book she received for Christmas. That's when you feel the loneliness of daddy's absence on Christmas day.

That's when reality set in that the most important wish on the Christmas list did not materialize—the one thing that was asked for every year for Christmas—DADDY! We never believed much in Santa Clause, but I (Tish) do remember seeing if he was real one year and if he could deliver the man of my dreams. Nope, Santa couldn't come through either.

I'm sure other children can relate to that experience of asking for something for Christmas and once you open all your gifts you realize you did not receive what you asked for and you don't give up expectations until the clock strikes 12:00 midnight. "Maybe mom and dad are going to surprise me with it much later", you think. We know that feeling. You check the garbage. Maybe it was accidentally thrown away. You circle the tree ten times. "It's got to be under this tree somewhere." You toss boxes around, shake gift bags, check the closets, search high and low— "This can't be right", you say. "That special gift I asked for has got to be around here somewhere."

That was how we felt year after year. Even after opening tens of awesome gifts, Christmas never felt complete without the presence of a father. It hurts when you see presents from mom and never anything from dad. It hurts that we never had that experience of shopping for something nice to buy daddy for Christmas. We will never know the look on his face as he opens that nice new necktie, or pair of argyle socks, or bottle of cologne. We will never know what that feels like to wrap a gift for daddy with a tag that says "To daddy, from your girls."

Birthdays were similar in terms of all-around fun and excitement during the day, met with an aching silence at day's end. To this day we still have most of the birthday cards we received from family members as keepsakes. Cards from grandparents, aunties, uncles, mom, siblings—so endearing. No cards from dad.

Birthdays were a big-time trigger for pain surrounding daddy. Birthdays are to celebrate your birth and entrance into the world. It's a day to receive lots of attention from loved ones as they celebrate your life. There would be no birthday for anyone without two parents coming together and procreating life. So, its understandable that birthdays were hard at times because the person who was key in the equation of procreating us was not in the picture.

Another important holiday that was a trigger for daddy hunger and stirred up hunger pangs was of course Father's Day. It's very difficult to forget you don't have a father on Father's Day. On this day young children and adult children can honor their fathers with gifts, cards, special words, shout outs, and countless other ceremonious dedications. It's a special holiday that designates time and opportunity to say "thank you" to dad and to celebrate all the fathers you know.

Many of these holidays were filled with sadness that we did not have a father of our own to honor or celebrate. Some were filled with gratitude for other males who filled in the gap. Yet some were experienced as "just another day" with feelings of indifference.

Milestones

Life is filled with various stages where a new skill is learned, where emotional, mental, and physical conditions advance to another major level, and where significant events occur. These are called milestones. Some of the most familiar developmental milestones occur before age 5 and include accomplishments like learning to smile socially, learning to crawl, learning to walk, and learning how to talk. These are undertakings that make caretakers/parents their absolute proudest and most joyous. As new parents ourselves, these are moments that we absolutely do not want to miss from our children.

A portion of our hunger pangs/pain comes from the knowledge that there was no proud papa in the picture to not only help us achieve these milestones but to cheer us on and celebrate that we "did it." There were no outstretched, strong, masculine arms to wobble to when we were learning how to walk. Learning to say "da-da" was irrelevant because it would never make the rotation of words in our vernacular. There would be no trip to the ice-cream shop as a reward from dad for reading our first complete sentence. No high-fives from daddy for going potty and no getting picked up and swung in the air to celebrate tying our shoes.

We didn't get our first bicycle until we were 13-14 years old for Christmas from an aunt of ours. They were very nice bikes, but we didn't know how to ride them. We were the only kids in our neighborhood that didn't know how to ride a bike and there was a degree of embarrassment about it. We had an open and unfinished basement at the time, so we would practice pedaling along the perimeter of the basement; using the wall to help stabilize us. There was one neighborhood friend named Bridgette who offered to help us learn, so when all the other kids were least likely to be outside, we would hang out with Bridgette and get some lessons. There was a small hill in our backyard and Bridgette said the best way to learn is to ride down the grassy hill. No pedaling was required just balancing, and once we had momentum on the flat foundation, we could let the bike coast and just maintain our balance until we were ready to pedal.

This technique worked like magic and didn't take long before we learned to ride those bikes. To accomplish something almost 10 years later than most kids, to skip training wheels, to overcome embarrassment and fear of falling, and mostly to do so without the craved support of dad was a huge deal. This was one of our most amazing milestones and one more great moment that was missing the presence of our father.

Accomplishments

We have accomplished a great deal in our lives both together and individually. You may be tired of hearing "we" so much throughout the book, but as identical twins we grew up being unusually close and linked together for just about everything we faced in at least 2/3 of our lives. So, yes, we were involved in much of the same activities, hobbies, and interests, however we differed in how we excelled through these involvements. There were many things that one was better at than the other and vice versa.

We did not have very many talents as children, at least none that were apparent or cultivated much. I'm sure we didn't always have the financial resources to at least go through the trial-and-error period where you help your children discover their talents. We were never athletic early on, but we started playing the violin in the 4th grade and stuck with it until we graduated high school. It was a nice skill to learn and grow into and we are grateful for the investment our mother made here. She supported us for many years and did a great job supporting us at our various events. It would have been nice to have daddy out in the audience as well at our various performances and concerts.

We were both shy as children, so we didn't participate in other performance-based activities. We did a little better than average academically and had various accomplishments in that area that it would have been nice to have daddy's smile of approval for, like making the honor roll or merit roll. We learned how to read around age 5 due to the diligence of one of our aunts making sure we made weekly trips to the neighborhood library. As grateful as we are for relatives filling in these gaps, there was still a longing in our hearts growing up for daddy to be there for us through these key accomplishments.

Another key accomplishment came in high school. We both tried out for the basketball team, and this is the perfect example of finding your true talent and skill by happenstance. We were horrible at basketball. We could not dribble. We could not ball-handle. We could not shoot. We were terribly uncoordinated for this sport. The only thing we were good at was running. We were fast and often we were ahead of everyone else during running drills.

Eventually the basketball coach pulled us both in his office to give us that dreaded talk—the one where a person tells you that your Option A goal is no longer an option for you and tries to persuade you to look at Option B. Well, he told us basketball was not working for us and offered for us to take stats instead. He also told us to try out for track since we were so fast. Well, we took his advice on both. We started working as the statisticians for the girls' basketball team and we also tried out for track and field our sophomore year of high school.

The failures in basketball lead to one of our biggest accomplishments as teens. We became valuable sprinters on our track team. We both ran the open 100-meter dash, the 200-meter dash, the 4 x 100 relay race, the 4 x 200 relay race and sometimes the open 400-meter race. We racked up lots of medals and accolades. We built a reputation along with our relay-team members in the city as a force to be reckoned with. People knew who we were before we knew them. Newspapers even made space for us in their sports sections. We broke a stadium record, which we heard is still unbeaten. Best of all, our relays landed us in the state track meet 2 years in a row. These were awesome years of success and achievement.

Our mother was super, duper supportive during our athletic success. She was at just about every one of our track and field meets and events cheering us on and letting everyone know around her that we were her precious daughters and she was so proud of us. This meant the world to us to have her there. She made sure we had the means to get whatever uniform and sports equipment we needed and made it to whatever practices we needed to. In addition to her, our extended family also was so proud and supportive of us.

As you can imagine, there was still a silent grief on the inside. A grief so heavy that no matter how many finish lines we crossed, no matter how many personal and stadium records we broke, no matter how many medals—we still wished dad was in the stands cheering for us. We still wish dad was there helping us carry our gym bags, patting us on the back and telling us to "go and get em" before our meets, and even making us finish our workouts when we slacked during practice and training (and boy did we slack a lot).

Other key accomplishments that we would have loved to have dad a part of were:

- High school graduation
- 1st day of college
- Salvation/Baptisms
- Learning to drive/getting driver's licenses
- Graduation from college
- First post-grad jobs
- Master's degrees
- Engagements
- Weddings
- Birth of children

Of this key list of accomplishments, you might be able to guess which ones stand out as most significant—you got it! Personal family goals and accomplishments!

Having a family of our own has always been one of our biggest desires in life and to be blessed with our own families is huge and noteworthy. From the first date all the way to the altar where vows were exchanged, these were seasons in our lives where we wish we had a dad around to share in the excitement and joy.

There is something special about taking "the one" home to meet your dad for the first time. Of all the achievements in life that you look forward to having your parents' approval of, certainly the mate that you choose is one of them. Had our father been in our lives, we know he would have been proud of our choices.

In both of our cases, our mates went to our mother to ask for our hands in marriage. This was very honorable, just atypical. And of course, when it came to deciding who would walk us down the aisle, we had to break tradition with that as well. Fatherlessness creates so many vacancies in every stage of life when you really do the math.

Which leads to the final major accomplishment we will explore which is having children. While we have accepted the reality that our children will probably never know their biological maternal grandfather, it still is upsetting, nevertheless. Our children's "normal" will include life without this paternal figure to share those classic memories with that most children get to experience.

If you're reading this and grew up with a father, we hope the accounts in this chapter brought light into the degree of hunger and the painfulness that we as fatherless daughters endured, the crisis it created and the crisis response needed, and the nutrients we often had to go without. If you walked in similar shoes to us, we hope this chapter validated some of your own experiences living with hunger pangs.

CHAPTER 4

THE FRAGMENTED BRAIN AND BODY

"Don't believe everything you hear –even in your own mind." –
Daniel Amen

"When you do not fully own your body, you cannot claim it for an
everlasting life."—Henri J.M. Nouwen

A little girl who is hungry for a dad and is lacking the nutrients that he often provides is at risk for having a fragmented mind and body. The mind and body are meant to receive nourishment—first in the home setting and then in alternate settings. Home is where most of the mealtimes occur, both natural meals and relational ones; waffles for breakfast with a side of wisdom—a ham sandwich for lunch with hugs—and spaghetti and spiritual guidance at night for dinner. Mealtimes are significant opportunities to be fed—and what a child is being fed at home determines how well he/she will function both in and outside of the home. In the previous chapter we talked about some important nutrients that fathers and mothers provide, and it is during "mealtimes" that these nutrients are served. So, you can see how important it is to have healthy adults in the home who know their roles as providers of these important mealtimes.

Our figurative mealtimes were a wee bit different due to not having a father in our lives. We had figures that provided us with appropriate nourishment for our young developing minds in our father's absence, but of course nothing can replace the role of a father. Our little minds were ready to soak up some major nutrients from daddy but ended up being met with hunger pangs and emptiness instead.

We know little kids are like sponges especially under the age of five. They soak up everything. That is awesome and scary at the same time. It's awesome because it denotes the power and learning capacity in children's brains. It is scary because this is the age range where children also soak up all the dysfunction, chaos, hurt, pain, wounds, and instability that may be found in their homes. This is such a critical age range for having the best nutrition, the best relational diet, and the healthiest consumption possible.

If nutrients are lacking, then there is a chance that the health of the mind will be compromised. In this chapter we will be exploring some of the functions of the mind and how daddy hunger impacted these functions in our lives and how a father's absence impacts the mind in general.

There is a statement that we learned in a grief group we participated in that said, "When your heart is broken, your head doesn't work!" Wow! How evident is that statement for anyone who has been through any kind of grief experience? Ever have a hard time concentrating after a break-up? Ever find yourself making bad decisions after a loss? Ever wonder why you can't process your emotions correctly after a painful rejection? It's because of the head injury that followed your heart injury! In other words, *Pain affects the Brain!*

There is a popular brain model in neuroscience research that explains the brain as being a 3-in-1 organ—it's called "The Triune Brain model" developed by Paul D. MacLean in 1990. This model posits that the brain was developed gradually in three parts starting from conception and completing in young adulthood. The building starts with the brain stem and cerebellum (The Body Brain), which is responsible for regulation of bodily functions like breathing, muscle control, regulating temperature, heart rate, sleep cycles, hunger and feeding cycles, bowel functioning and arousal. Then the Limbic System (The Emotion Brain) develops next, which is the center for emotions, a monitor of danger and safety, where attachment and sense of smell are, where escape plans like fight or flight originate from and where positive and negative memories are encoded. Next, the Neocortex (The Thinking Brain) is developed which is responsible for higher order thinking and executive functioning skills like planning, logic, reflection, imagination, predictions, decision-making, empathy, and language.

So, when we say a broken heart caused our heads to malfunction, we mean our brain stem, limbic brain, and neocortex were affected—our bodily functions that flow from the brain, our feelings and our thinking were wounded. Throughout this chapter, we will explore exactly how pain affected our brains and maybe you will see how your pain may have affected your brain too.

THE BODY BRAIN

The lack of a quality attachment figure had some minor interference with how our base brains functioned. Remember the base brain or brain stem is responsible for basic bodily functions. It may seem like a stretch to believe that there could even be such an unusual connection between relational pain and the brain in this way, but our experiences really do interact with our mind and body in fascinating ways.

It's not that hard to believe that you don't sleep very well when your heart is broken—and sleep cycles come out of the brain stem. Sometimes thinking too much about our absent father caused us to want to sleep excessively and sometimes not at all. We both were diagnosed with sleep disorders in our 20s and still suffer to various degrees with sleep dysfunction, which includes an REM sleep disorder. REM sleep disorder symptoms include excessive time spent in REM stage of sleep, as well as movements and talking in sleep. We also experience frequent disturbing dreams about childhood and our childhood homes.

Pain interferes with your ability to regulate hunger and feeding cycles. There were times of mourning our childhood when we experienced a loss of appetite followed by over-eating or emotional eating. There were plenty of times where we really weren't physically hungry—we were relationally hungry. Hunger signals don't come from the stomach or brain stem with emotional eating, the signals come from the emotional brain.[1] It wasn't necessarily a physical hunger that took a toll on us; it was the hunger in our limbic brain that took a toll. We were stuffing donuts in our mouths, not in response to a growling tummy; but in response to a growling heart that just wanted a dad (but those donuts were still yummy).

Other ways we noticed brain stem dysfunction was in our breathing patterns. We both have struggled to regulate our breathing properly. Our breathing styles range from holding our breath to hyperventilating if we are not mindful of practicing proper breathing techniques. We both also have learned where we hold our fatherlessness stories in our muscular tissues. Our muscle imbalances can be attributed to our feelings of loss, despair, shame, and stored fears. Emotions affect muscle tone.[2] I (Tish) hold a lot of tension in my shoulders, throat, back and abdominal muscles. I (Nell) hold a lot of my tension in my back, jaws, hips, and chest. We both have learned ways to address our muscular systems and bring them back to harmony, ease, and coordination.

As we share some ways that our body brains became fragmented, in what ways are you more curious about how your breathing, sleep, eating, muscular and bowel and bladder systems function because of your story?

THE EMOTION BRAIN

There is a significant impact of fatherlessness and daddy hunger on this part of the brain. Social and emotional intelligence are primary functions of this area of the brain, but this development can be grossly interrupted if there are significant attachment disruptions. Emotions can be dysregulated and disproportionate, attachment experiences are logged in the brain under the "insecure" tab, emotional memories are stored here, and problems occur with properly interpreting threats and safety.

Due to the lack of our father and not having such an important familial figure in our lives, our overall emotional well-being was fragmented and malnourished! We did not cope well with minor or major changes in life. We were often overly fearful and anxious. We also dealt with extremes of being overly attached to certain things or people. We can recall many occasions where we cried because of trivial reasons. Some examples involve crying when people left us temporarily, on last days of school, if we had to stop playing for the night, or if we lost pieces of paper with notes on them. We just could not handle normal day-to-day transitions, the crossing of thresholds and changes. Our emotions were starving for the vitamins and minerals that can only come from constant positive input and support from a father.

THE THINKING BRAIN

The very sophisticated and most complex of all the three brains is the neocortex. It is in the uppermost part of the brain and toward the front behind your forehead. Even the placement of this distinguished part of the brain suggests that its use helps us to Think Up and move up and out from other regions of the brain where we often get stuck or flooded. At the top is where we have the most clarity and access to wisdom and truth. We communicate better, we make better decisions, and we can direct and lead other parts of who we are effectively. But this part of the brain is at risk for fragmenting when faced with attachment trauma. One way that this fragmentation manifests is through negative thinking habits.

Stinkin' Thinkin'

Stinkin' Thinkin' is a psychological term to describe distortions in one's thinking. These distortions of thought cause one to believe they will fail, that bad things will happen to them or that they are not a very good person. When a person's thinking is distorted, it causes distortions in feelings and behavior. There are tons of books out there from both Christian and secular perspectives on the idea of improving thinking—and these books tend to fly off the shelves. Research proves that improved thinking improves the way a person feels, and who doesn't want to feel better? The key to feeling better is confronting, challenging, and changing distorted or stinkin' thinkin'.

When you hear the phrase stinkin' thinkin', it almost makes you want to plug your nose. What kind of thinking would make someone want to plug his or her nose? Food that stinks indicates it may be spoiled or expired. It has exceeded its ability to maintain its freshness. So, it probably won't be very nutritious to consume. Thoughts that stink have lost their freshness. They are rotten and are not healthy for your mind to consume.

Furthermore, when a thought is distorted, it means that thought has deviated from the truth. The truth is what keeps our minds fresh and healthy. Thoughts that are not based on the truth begin to carry an odor—and an odorous mind is not appealing. The Bible is a great source of truth for us to feed our minds with. There are many scriptures that highlight God and His word as vital nutrients of truth for our minds:

"Jesus answered, 'I am the way, and the truth, and the life. No one comes to the Father except through me'" (John 14:6 NIV)

"Then you will know the truth, and the truth will set you free." (John 8:32 NIV)

"You belong to your father, the devil, and you want to carry out your father's desires. He was a murderer from the beginning, not holding to the truth, for there is no truth in him. When he lies, he speaks his native language, for he is a liar and the father of lies." (John 8:44 NIV)

"God is not human, that he should lie." (Numbers 23:19 NIV)

"All your words are true; all your righteous laws are eternal." (Psalm 119:160 NIV)

"Sanctify them by the truth; your word is truth." (John 17:17 NIV)

"Guide me in your truth and teach me." (Psalm 25:5 NIV)

"Teach me your way, O Lord; I will walk in your truth." (Psalm 86:11 NASB)

Of course, these are just a few passages that emphasize the beauty of knowing Christ and the truth He offers us. Once you embrace the reality that God cannot lie and that everything He has ever said is true, then you can find Him and His word to be 100% trustworthy. The truth does so much for the wellbeing of our hearts and minds and is the remedy for any distorted thoughts that we have. According to scripture, distortions in thinking are not from God. Distorted thoughts keep us bound. His desire is for us to be led in truth and to be free. Anything that we think and believe about ourselves that is not grounded in God's truth is technically a lie, and lies come from the father of lies—Satan! And we know he is incapable of telling the truth and only capable of *stinkin' thinkin'*!

These realizations were so critical for us in our journey growing up without a father, because although our feelings were wounded, we did not want our thinking to be a source of lies. When your situation is bad, it is very easy to begin to think bad thoughts—thoughts that stink. We were both guilty of stinkin' thinkin' and entertaining rotten, spoiled, and decayed thoughts about being fatherless. John Bradshaw states that a common thought distortion of those with father wounds is "If my father abandons me, all men will abandon me."[3] Have you ever battled an overgeneralized thought like that? Here are some distorted thoughts about fatherlessness that we had to confront, and you may have had to in your journey:

- I'm an accident!
- Not having a father is the worst!
- God is not good!
- I am alone!
- God doesn't love me!
- How could God do this?
- Why me?
- I'll never heal!
- I can't get past this!
- Will I ever find true love?
- I'm unlovable!
- I'm forgotten!
- I'm left out!
- I must be a bad person!
- I'm damaged goods!
- I'll have a bad life!
- There's no way I'll survive this!
- My past defines me and controls my destiny!

It can be quite automatic to resort to stinkin' thinkin', not because you wanted to think that way, but because your mind was trying to make sense of the broken pieces of your life—you couldn't quite land on the truth and instead ended up in a pile of lies. We couldn't find the truth about the good that would come out of growing up without a father and so we repeatedly wrestled with painful thoughts instead. These thoughts occurred somewhere in between the lemons and the lemonade.

Some, not all, of our painful and odorous thoughts evolved into personal truths. We really began to believe some of our laments. What you believe in can be either a blessing or a burden to you. If what you believe about yourself and your situation is not "true", then that is a very dangerous belief. Nothing or no one can convince you otherwise. When what you believe is the truth, according to God's word, then you are in the right position to receive blessing upon blessing. The times we held on to the false-truth that we were unlovable, we were in the danger zone and had a hard time believing anyone or anything that suggested otherwise—at times even God's word seemed to smack right into the wall of the lies we held on to.

Purposeful vs Problematic Questions

Some smelly thoughts are in the form of exclamations or statements, and some are questions. Sometimes we don't realize that the questions we pose in our minds—pose a problem!

There is a major difference between a problematic question and a purposeful one. When we ask questions in our minds, they will fall under one of the two categories. It's all about intent! When your intention is for your question to be a starting point that directs you to truth then you are on the right path. When your questions lead you right back to the dump you started at, then your question was more of a set up for more harm. Let's look at some examples of purposeful vs problematic questions:

Problematic question: How could God do this?
Purposeful question: What might God's purpose be in allowing this?

Problematic question: Why me?
Purposeful question: How can I grow from this?

Problematic question: Will I ever find love?
Purposeful question: What things can I do now to love myself?

These are examples of how you can shift your mind into reframing problematic questions into questions that are more likely to lead you to helpful insights, revelations, and self-growth.

Self-Reflection

Self-reflection is an important function of the neocortex. When this part of the brain is functioning at its best, a person can peer inward and evaluate what is going on in the inner-most parts. Knowing what is going on in the inner-most parts helps to regulate what manifests on the outer-most parts. The outward is what people see and how people experience you. The outward tends to be behavioral traits. In most cases, the better the ability to self-reflect, the better the behavior and attitude!

When this part of the brain is functioning at its worst, then you can expect self-reflection and personal insights to be limited and flawed. If your self-reflection is poor, you can expect to be the last to know you have issues. Everyone sees your issues but you. This may be because you lack the time to sit and go inward or you lack the skills. Self-reflection requires being able to both push pause on life and ask the right questions. Unfortunately, pain gets in the way of one's ability to stop and ask the right questions.

Self-reflection is so important and vital to healthy relationships. It is very burdensome on those you love when they must constantly be the ones to tell you about your inappropriate or offensive behavior and attitudes. It drains those relationships and puts all the pressure on loved ones to be the ones to inform you about how you are behaving. This also increases the chances of there being defensiveness if you are on the receiving end of outside information about your behavior.

It is much more ideal to be able to ascertain what your issues are by way of taking time to reflect. Change often is more meaningful when you take stock of your own areas of self-improvement and then make personal commitments to change in those areas. It is very humbling to be honest with yourself during those "ah hah" moments. There is an expression that the hardest person to be honest with is the person you see in the mirror. We find this expression to be true!

Now everyone has blind spots; issues to which no matter how much self-reflection you do, you are just likely to overlook. We need others to reflect to us what is going on so we can consider improvement. It is also very humbling (or embarrassing) to have someone point out your flaws or blind spots. It is obvious that you are cared for deeply when someone comes to you about something you are doing (of course we don't always receive it as such). Having others point out your blind spots can be very healthy for relationships; however, others' reflection does not take the place of self-reflection.

Because of our daddy-pain, sometimes we have fallen short in our ability to self-reflect and evaluate our own issues. Truth is, we both have deep issues, some of which have interfered with our ability to have: 1) Healthy relationships and 2) Healthy interactions in past & current relationships.

There is a difference between having failed relationships and having failed interactions within healthy relationships. Our inabilities to self-reflect led to several failed or unhealthy relationships, but it also led to frequent unhealthy choices within healthy relationships.

We have been guilty of allowing our pain to cloud our insight and other times we have had an attitude of entitlement to our issues—almost as if to say, "I'm allowed to have these issues since I don't have a dad" or "With all I've been through, I deserve to act a little crazy sometimes and people need to just deal." These attitudes of entitlement are wrong!

We have had our share of others coming to us to point out areas of growth, whether these "others" were family, friends, mentors, leaders, supervisors, or our spouses. And it is indeed very humbling and even hurtful at times. It's humbling because it gives you the opportunity to apologize in those moments and seek reparation. It can be hurtful because you realize your actions have affected others and you truly never wanted that to happen. And if we are honest, our pride gets a little bruised.

Confronting our issues with self-reflection has been an important part of our holistic care routines. Individually, we both have set up habits of journaling, having quiet time, asking pertinent questions, looking for growth areas, and then making steps to change. There are plenty of areas where we've seen long-term healing while there are other areas we've had difficulty seeing effective improvement. But we know the more we reflect inward, the more those stuck areas are going to have to shift in the direction of healing.

Emotion Processing

The neocortical region of the brain, when at its optimal functioning, is responsible for processing through emotions that come out of the limbic brain in an adaptive way. Emotion processing means to be inquisitive of your emotions so that you can understand them better. Once you understand them better, you can heal them. It also can mean seeing emotions through to resolution.

Emotions are powerful messengers that:

- Inform us of what is happening around us

- Alert us to significant details in our environments

- Inform us of who or what is safe vs. unsafe

- Notify us of our needs and how those needs are being met

- Flag if we are getting too much of something or not enough

- Prompt us to an action we need to take

- In and of themselves are neither good nor bad

So, if these are some key functions of emotions, then emotion processing would mean finding out what the message is that the messenger is delivering by answering questions like these below:

- What is the emotion?

- What is this emotion trying to alert me to?

- What is happening that triggered this feeling? What has occurred in the past 24 hours?

- Is the person I'm interacting with a safe person (emotionally and/or physically)? Is this situation safe?

- What am I aware of that I need right now? Is this need getting met?

- What am I getting too much of? What am I not getting enough of?

- What action do I need to take? What conversation do I need to have?

By the time you answer some of these questions, you should have a better understanding of the presenting emotion(s) and have some direction for what to do next to adaptively resolve what you are feeling. Oh wait, that sounds good on paper, but in practice, it can be very hard to resolve what you feel.

This has often been our sentiment growing up with daddy-hunger. Father pain makes the brain go haywire. Emotions are muddled and processing is fuddled. It has been very difficult to make sense of the cocktail of emotions and thread-by-thread untangle the interwoven yarn-ball of feelings. There has often been a desperation followed by exasperation at every attempt to resolve the chaos in our limbic brains. "Where do I start? Which emotion do I even fix first? I'm too exhausted from pain to even sort this all out! This is going to take a lifetime to figure out! Is this even humanly possible to feel 20 emotions at once? Is there even a word in the English language to define this emotion I feel? I must be crazy to even feel this way! Where's the off switch?"

Does this emotional tirade sound familiar to you? This has unmusically played out in our heads too many times to count. This is what failure to process looks like. It's when you don't know where to start so you plop down, cross your arms, and say, "No way!" It's much easier to drown in the lake of painful emotions then to get out the emotional processing floatation devices and seek safety. That's what daddy-hunger does—you're so hungry for daddy that you can't calm your limbic brain down enough to make your way to the front of your head to sort through what you feel. You're literally "stuck in the middle." If you've ever gone too long without eating, you know it's much more difficult to process your feelings than if you've had 3 square meals—in that case you were stuck in your brain stem or bottom brain. So, like being "stuck in the bottom" when you've skipped too many meals—daddy-hunger is being stuck in another part of the brain that keeps you from processing.

Wisdom, Judgement and Decision-Making

If we had a nickel for every foolish idea we've had or choice we've made, we could retire early! Well...maybe that's an exaggeration but we would have a lot of nickels. The truth is this function of our brain stayed relatively intact. We've always had a degree of gifting in the wisdom department throughout our formative years. Even throughout adulthood, we have seen our gifts of discernment blossom and grow. But there are notable times, mostly during hetero-gender relationship experiences where our wisdom has suffered the most.

Trying to manage relationships "wisdom-impaired" is a recipe for disaster! Another awesome word for wisdom is sapience. It's a cool word derived from the Latin word sapientia, which means wisdom. If you've ever taken a human evolution class or an anthropology class in college, you may have even heard of the term homo sapiens coined by Carl Linnaeus to describe human beings, which he came up with to denote the unique difference between humans and animals—the gift of wisdom! While we do not believe in evolution, we do believe wisdom is what sets us apart from all other creatures that God created. But sometimes in relationships, we didn't live up to these expectations—we behaved in ways a bit more like our animal friends. We allowed sheer attraction to determine which male species to give our phone number to, we froze in fear when we should've had boundaries, we submitted to male species we should have ran from, we migrated with herds we shouldn't have, and we allowed our hunger for daddy to cause us to pounce on males at times demanding they feed us much deserved love, commitment, and affection—you know?—all things that animals who lack wisdom do. We were wisdom-impaired at times for sure!

Our definition of having a wisdom-impairment is:

- A lack of understanding regarding how male-female relationships work

- Having opaque discernment about men's character

- Not balancing the gift of circumspection well; either being too cautious or not cautious enough, too guarded, and not guarded enough, too suspicious, or not suspicious enough

- An inadequate use of common-sense

- Allowing interest to over-ride intuition

- Allowing mating-instincts to override gut-instincts

We also suffered from judgment-impairments as well. There is a slight difference between wisdom and judgment. Wisdom is the insight into what is right and what is wrong; judgment is that action, choice or result of the wisdom.

Our definition of having a judgment-impairment is:

- Failing to learn from some relationship mistakes and repeating them

- Proceeding after recognizing red flags

- Giving males access to us after our guts told us "No"

- Doing the opposite of what we believed was best

- Our actions contradicting our deepest convictions

- Following impulses and acting without thinking

- Saying "yes" too often and to the wrong people

We are not 100% convinced that having a father would have spared us these various malnourishments in our thinking brains, but we are confident that the right doses of the right nutrients from a healthy father would have given our brains quite a boost in the wisdom department when it came to interacting with the opposite sex.

Logic and Meaning-Making

When navigating relationships with daddy-hunger, it can sometimes be hard to connect the dots and make connections with the limited information people often give to you about themselves. People and relationships can be quite a puzzle; you get bits and pieces of who people are and you try your best to put it all together so you can determine if this person is a good fit to be in your life.

But even with all the dots that you must connect, sometimes its ridiculously obvious which relationships are safe and appropriate and which ones are not. It's logical. No deep discernment is needed. No gut responses required. No visions and dreams needed to give you insight into the person you are dealing with. Just logic. And you know which gender tends to be more logical? You got it—men!

Growing up we wished we had a logical fatherly perspective on how to handle relationships. If a guy we liked and who seemed to like us too went days, weeks, months without calling, we struggled to connect the dots and make sense about what that meant. "Does he like me or not?" was a frequent question in our minds. We were waiting on some super meaningful wisdom about it—when really it was quite simple—when a guy likes you, he calls you—EVERYDAY! We wished we could have had "dad" investing this kind of logic into us as we grew up. We imagine him saying, "Daughters, if a guy likes you, he will call! He's not calling for a very simple reason—he's just not into you so let him go!"

Logic means sometimes seeing things for what they are. It means seeing the relationship between cause and effect. Many times, we saw things for what we wanted them to be instead of what they really were. Logic means "1+1=2." We could have saved ourselves from a lot of heartbreak had we done the simple math. Simple math means, if you want a guy who is a great conversationalist but the guy you are head-over-heels about only sends one-word text responses when you reach out to him and doesn't elaborate when you talk on the phone, then he's not the right guy for you. We hungered for a dad who could teach us these simple logical truths in dating.

Meaning-making is also crucial and an important function of the thinking brain. It's another way to connect the dots as you navigate life. It's the ability to a) produce a thesis out of a whole story and b) understand the rationale for the way things are. It's the ability to answer the questions of "how & why."

There's an awesome quote that states, "Suffering ceases to be suffering the moment you obtain a meaning." That's profound, isn't it? Is this saying that most of our suffering is because we don't know the answers to "why" we go through various storms? Is this supposing that most of our grief is because we don't know the meaning or purpose of the loss? Hmm! We would argue that a meaning could afford a sufferer a great deal of healing in their journey, but there will likely be deposits of pain leftover no matter what.

For us, we didn't have the skills to make sense of our circumstance in our formative years. In fact, things didn't make sense for a long time. No bachelor's degree and no master's degree could provide us with the proficiency to make a meaning out of our family predicament. There was just no reasonable explanation for why we didn't have a father. Our minds were truly malnourished!

It would take years of hard work and healing before we would even have a workable theory. Our workable theory for many years was

"God has a purpose and a plan for this pain and something good will come out of it."

This reads in a very abstruse way. It sounds good and yet very mysterious at the same time. We couldn't know for sure what good would come out of it, we just had to believe. We didn't know for certain the purpose, but we had to believe anyway. This meaning-making affirmation doesn't directly or explicitly provide the clearest meaning for "Why don't I have a father?" But it expands the heart and mind to explore the deeper meaning and we will reveal to you what we've learned a little later about the meaning of being fatherless.

Language Limitations

The last function of the thinking brain we will share with you is weighty. There is no doubt that when it comes to the malnourished mind, this faculty of our heads suffered a great starvation. Our ability to express ourselves through the gift of language is unequivocally one of the most damaged parts of our minds.

Language is an important part of the neocortical regions of the brain, specifically, the Broca's area. Broca's area was discovered by brain surgeon Paul Broca and has been scientifically linked to speech production and language processing in the brain. Physical injuries to the front region of the brain could damage this region, but we are not talking about a physical injury that caused our language limitations. We also are not talking about a speech disorder that would warrant the attention of a speech therapist. What we are speaking of is a relational-emotional-social wounding that happened to our brains because of our pain, where we failed to learn to use our voices with people.

We grew up in a home and culture where a child's voice was not valued highly. We grew up under the legacy burden passed down from generation to generation that "children are to be seen and not heard." We are early 80's babies, so this family commandment is not surprising if you grew up in a similar or even earlier era. While we hold no ill-will toward those who imposed this commandment on us through words, through actions, or attitudes, we wish we were never taught such a damaging rule. This rule threatened to strip our voices away from us forever.

What people who teach this rule fail to understand is that, while you may mean for this rule to just apply to home-life, it breaks those bounds and affects the social-life, love-life, job-life, church-life, ministry-life, spouse-life—and any other kind of environment where your child needs their voice. The "children are not to be heard" rule is one of the foulest rules ever and should be banned from every home and from the human vocabulary. The no-feel rule and the no-talk rule are two common rules in dysfunctional families.[4]

There were also similar messages regarding our voices that we internalized. There was one occasion where we were speaking up passionately about something to a family member, and this individual responded that we didn't have wisdom because essentially only the adults in the family have wisdom—another legacy burden and wound to our already wounded voices.

Other ways we feel our voices became wounded and starved were:

- Being dismissed when we expressed ourselves (i.e. lack of response, changing the subject, being told to be quiet, being told we were being disrespectful)

- Primary figures failing to ask us our thoughts, feelings, opinions about things

- Being talked at versus talked to

- Being cut off or over-talked when we did share

- When approaching adults with calm, quiet voices being matched with loud and aggressive voices

- When trying to share our hearts and we were met with over-spiritualization to dismiss our thoughts and feelings

These wounding agents had long lasting impact on us in our relationships and in various environments where we truly needed strong, well-nourished voices and instead were left with weak, depleted vocalizations. Many of our hurts in relationships have been due to our inability to speak up for ourselves, establish boundaries with others vocally, and say no when needed. We have often frozen in place (there's that animal response again), when it came to sharing our thoughts, feelings, and opinions with others, even to the present. Fear has taken over one-too-many times when it was time to speak. We have swallowed a lot of our own words that should have been released. We have choked and gagged on valuable communications because of awful lies in our head that told us "We are only to be seen and not heard." Swallowing so many words didn't add any pounds to our souls, because when words are meant to be released and you swallow them, it's like taking in poison that eats away at whatever good you have stored inside. It's through using your voice that you actually "get gains" as they say in the fitness world.

Voice wounds can also manifest into a clinical disorder of social anxiety. Pertinent symptoms related to the use of the voice are:

- A trembling or shaky voice

- Avoiding speaking to people out of fear of embarrassment

- Intense fear of talking or interacting with others

- Expecting the worst consequences out of social situations (sharing your thoughts)

- In severe cases, a choking anxiety or choking sensation that presents when it's time to talk in certain situations

We think you understand a little better about our voice wounds, but what do these language wounds have to do with being fatherless? In a healthy home environment, a father helps his daughter to find her voice and use it in a healthy way. A lot of this is modeled through how the father uses his own voice in the home. Men typically have naturally powerful and influential voices. They often teach their children how to stand up for themselves, how to speak their convictions with passion, how not to take no for an answer (when this approach is warranted), how to be confident in what they think and feel and how to speak clearly and be fearless in communication.

It would be a stretch to say we would have been guaranteed these skills had we had a father, but we truly believe the lack of a consistent and healthy male voice in our environment provided us with little to no nutrients to even build off. But there is hope!

God Restores Broken Voices

There are two voice types we will review that we have identified with because of our malnourished minds and two restored voice types that are the outcome of healing. We believe God can heal any language limitation and restore the broken voice no matter what the cause.

The Victim Voice

This voice says, "I am not worthy to be listened to" and "No one cares about what I have to say." So, it stays quiet and remains a victim to the voices around it. This voice submits to all other voices around it. The best way to get along with others is to allow others' thoughts, feelings, and opinions to dominate the conversation.

The Violent Voice

This voice was once a victim, and to compensate for being a victim, it says, "Everyone will hear me now." "I have a lot to say, and I don't care who I hurt." This voice injures people with the things that it says to get power back from all the times it was the victim voice. This voice shouts, is angry, is aggressive, is overly opinionated and charges its way through conversations. One of the biggest excuses the violent voice uses is "Well other people took my voice away." Or "I just want to be heard."

Jesus came to heal these voices and turn them into voices that are valued and voices that are victorious.

The Valued Voice

This voice believes it has value; therefore, it is free to share and communicate without bowing to apprehension or blurting out abuse. It does not operate out of fear, nor does it need to create fear in others. Confidence is the attitude this voice utilizes each time it communicates. This voice doesn't have anything to prove and is not trying to even the score, even though it's suffered its share of "shh-shing." The value this voice carries doesn't come from others' appreciation of it; it comes from the godly approval from above and within.

The Victorious Voice

This voice has suffered years of "hushing" and has been broken and beaten down by others, but it has risen from the ashes. This voice has used its years of being lost to help others find their lost voices. This voice goes beyond victories in everyday communication and has used its gift to communicate healing to others specifically through verbal means or public speaking. This voice had a purpose to be heard and has the attitude, "Because I was told to be quiet, I am going to share my voice with the world."

If like us, you have lost your voice along the way, never learned how to use it, or feel fatherlessness has put you at a disadvantage with the utilization of your voice, here are some steps you can take to gain nourishment:

- Write down every ill-spoken opinion and lie you've been told regarding your voice and hold your own burial/release ceremony

- Write down 5-10 truths about your voice & read them often

- Find & memorize scripture that emphasize the power of your voice

- Take a communications skills course

- Seek out a Christian counselor

- Practice using your voice in prayer

- Take time for weekly self-reflection

- Build a circle of safe ears to share with; remove people who constantly shame your voice

- Practice talking in a mirror

THE FRAGMENTED BODY

We have talked about some of the functions of the body as it relates to the brain stem. We will go into more detail about the connection between fatherlessness and the soma here. Soma is the Greek word for body.[5] The body reacts and responds to what is going on in the environment around it in so many ways that are both instinctual and creative. We believe the body is wise and sacred and knows how to heal. Even under attack, the body is meant to do what it can to survive. The body speaks, communicates, alerts, and moves in and out of various states in a transient way as a part of normal functioning.

So, when we speak of a fragmented body, we are not necessarily stating that the body is an enemy that needs to be criticized and conquered. The body has just become disorganized and detached—within systems, organs, tissues, nerves and how it moves and functions. The body is at war with disturbances and needs compassion and friendship. The fragmenting becomes a problem when we won't draw close to the body, get curious about it and how it reacts to stress, and start to help it unburden and become united.

One way that broken hearts turns into fragmented bodies is through somatic dissociation. A simple definition of Somatic Dissociation according to Zimberoff and Hartman, is parts of the body that do not feel.[6] We also understand dissociation to be a way the body fragments within itself; cutting off conscious awareness. We cannot care for what we do not feel!

Our father hunger caused disruption in how we paid attention to our bodies, how we listened to the story our bodies had to tell, how we connected with our bodies and our capacity to be more embodied.

What is Embodiment? It is "feeling oneself directly, without the constant narration or interpretation of our thinking mind."[7] Embodiment is so important because we were created to be one with our bodies. But somehow, we have moved away from being human beings to human doings. As a culture, we cannot tolerate the stillness that we need and inappropriately call it boredom which leads us to over-entertaining ourselves with media and devices. We need to move back towards being-ness and not doing-ness.

Fatherlessness is such a profound trauma that it can lead to severe fragmentation and disembodiment. Moving from disembodiment to embodiment is attainable simply by bringing more awareness to your body, spending more time in nature, breathwork, healthy touch, engaging in curative movement practices or being more present with yourself.

CHAPTER 5

THE HUNGRY HEART

"My flesh and my heart may fail, but God is the strength of my heart and my portion forever." (Psalm 73:26 NASB)

"Many of the expressions of hunger we experience as adults have their roots in a childhood feeling, experience, fear, or hurt. They are the result of a wound that never healed."
—Robin Smith

Our lives and our hearts are literally filled with a huge empty space. We have a major void that cannot be denied or discounted no matter how badly our minds want us to just move on. It goes back to the scenario of an empty stomach that growls and contracts to alert the person that hunger is apparent and needs to be dealt with. The stomach has such a void that even if several hours go by with no food, the stomach's plea for food is not going to cease. Hunger comes with being human and hunger unattended is a tormenter.[1] The same is true for the hungry heart waiting for the love of a father to fill it. There may be some moments where the hunger pangs rest, but they always come back—always!

VOID FILLERS

Voids are real—they are not imagined! An empty refrigerator is void of food. An empty gas tank is void of fuel. An empty pool is void of water. When God created the world, He specifically stated that the earth was null and void; formless and empty (See Genesis 1:1-2). Acknowledging emptiness or a void is not claiming defeat or that all hope is lost. It is simply being aware that something is missing or "not there." Whether the void can or even should be filled is subjective. In our case, we have gone through many seasons of either trying to fill our void or just letting it be.

We mentioned earlier how even in our daily diets, we sometimes fill the void of hunger with unhealthy snacks or items specifically marketed to be meal replacements, like shakes or protein bars. The purpose of most snacks or small meal replacements is to "tie a person over." We have all heard and used the phrase "I just need something to tie me over" and we know the purpose is not usually long-term fulfillment, but short-term. The problem with "tie-me-overs" is they only last so long and without sufficient nutrients, another "tie-me-over" will be needed just to carry on.

It is safe to say that we have lived much of our lives with the "tie-me-over" mentality. We have craved and salivated for quick fixes and void-fillers to heal our hungry hearts, and none have sufficed. What we had to learn as we matured is nothing—nothing can truly satiate the yearning of a father. If a person goes a day without a real meal, the chips, granola, or soda will be minimally satisfying. We have listed some snacks and void fillers that we used at one point or another to attempt to fill our father-void:

- Music
- Sugar (not just sugary foods, but actual white granulated sugar)
- Junk food or comfort food
- Toys, excessive child's play
- Drawing/Coloring
- Masturbation
- Isolating
- Writing
- Sleep
- Silliness, excessive laughing and joking
- Church, religion
- Work
- Shopping/Spending Money
- Sex/Sexual-related experiences

- Collecting Items (rocks, paper, sea-shells, clothes, shoes, etc)

- Fantasizing

- People (friends, co-workers, mentors, church affiliates, pastors)

- Busyness

These void-fillers have each been used at some point in our lives from early childhood all the way to adulthood. Many of these were insatiable cravings, some were even ingestive addictions or oral fixations, like our struggle with emotional and compulsive eating. These behaviors are symptoms of what Fritz Perls calls a Growth Disorder; they formed out of the void created by unmet needs.[2]

Before we look specifically at our void-fillers, let's define what hunger looks like — It's a deep longing and a need to be truly known, accepted, respected, loved, valued, seen, and heard by the self and others. When hunger is neglected, ignored, denied, shamed, blamed, or misunderstood it makes us even hungrier. The more we deny our hunger pains, the stronger our cravings become, leading us to act out destructively — because hungry people do desperate things. This desperation might be manifested in overachieving, underachieving, depression, false elation, seeking power, becoming powerless, being a victim, being a victimizer, or having emotional and/or sexual affairs. Hunger has many faces, but one way or another it demands to be fed.[3]

Here are some of the void-fillers we have used:

People

People were very popular void-fillers for our hungry hearts. Unfortunately, some people were poisonous or toxic to us, but we couldn't discriminate this at the time because we were so empty inside. We experienced what R.T. Kendall calls pseudo-guilt, which is the affective response that occurred whenever we filled up on stuff we didn't really enjoy, like pain and maltreatment because we wanted to people-please.[4] It's as if we allowed people to force a fork of something undesirable in our mouths and we chewed it with hesitation and choked it down forcefully.

We tolerated unhealthy relationships to save face and in turn, we suffered. We suffered because we didn't like the pain of hunger.

We also tended to be gullible, naïve, and passive in certain relationships, or what John Bradshaw says is a tendency to "swallow things whole."[5] This is not a surprise when it comes to hunger. Hungry people don't always chew their food thoroughly and often take in too much food at one time instead of taking small, manageable bites.

Shopping

Shopping was another major void-filler. We loved to go to Target in our early college days and spend our hard-earned work-study money. If we saw a cute purse, pair of shoes, or pajamas, we just had to have it. I mean, who can resist those alluring colors and those red clearance stickers at Target? It felt like an addiction sometimes. If we had $231.00 in our shared account, we would reason that we could spend exactly $228.00 and be okay.

Who could possibly be sad when they have a white and red bag full of chic, adorable shirts, and cropped pants? We would get back to our dorm room and unpack our bags excitedly and rip the tags off our new purchases and store the items away because we knew they were for keeps. Never ever would we return anything. Even while being so excited to put away our purchases, we were fearful and would cringe to balance our checkbook seeing that we had two to three dollars left in our account. Unfortunately, that fear of being low on money was not enough for us to humbly pack up our purchases and drive them back to the store.

We just wanted to feel filled up. And if being broke was the temporarily price to pay for that filled-up feeling, then we gladly accepted the consequences. Many of you can relate to using shopping or other fillers to try and rid yourself of pain. We did not know exactly why we were grieving at times or what we were hungry for, but we were filling a void. Have you ever been so hungry that you felt you could eat anything, but when you opened the refrigerator, you just stood there confused? Or if someone asked you what you had a taste for, you responded that you did not know? Well, we lived much of our lives being hungry for a father but did not know that is what we were hungry for. So, we shopped and made other careless choices in life because we were looking to fill a void but did not know what we truly wanted. We wanted something to make the hunger go away, we just did not choose healthy options at times.

Sleep

Another void-filler that we just must unpack is sleeping. Ahh—we can just feel the coolness of the pillow and soft bed now! Sleeping is scientifically and biologically meant to offer restoration and serves as a reboot for the entire body. Every human and even animals need a daily sleep regimen to maintain a healthy and balanced life. However, sleep can serve as a get-a-way, an addiction, or in our case a void-filler. There is a healthy amount of sleep that is required for each individual and that amount is different from person to person. For us, there have been many instances where sleep went well beyond healthy to an obsession.

Many times, we were not even sleepy or tired, yet we still decided to force ourselves to take a nap or sleep-in well into noon. We must add a plug in here and say that we both have suffered with sleeping disorders throughout our adulthood so that is a factor in why our sleep cycles are not the greatest, but we are still aware that we used sleep as a drug in many cases. There are some points in life where things were just bleak and troublesome and sleeping was the antidote to dealing with pressures of life.

Sleep was literally a mini vacation away from troublesome thoughts, problems, and life battles that we just did not want to face. The problem with using sleep as a vacation is as soon as you wake up, the problem is still there. There is no true escape from life's challenges. And certainly, there is no escape from missing your biological father. The best nap in the world cannot fill the void or take away the pain of an absent father. Sleep, like many other void-fillers is like pulling a beautiful area rug over a gaping hole in the floor hoping that the hole isn't noticeable. Unfortunately, that hole is still very much a nuisance and puts one at risk for a great fall.

What void-fillers have you used in your life to cope with the chronic emptiness from a missing father?

BINGEING ON BOYS

Boys, boys, boys! The unreasonable crushes and unintentional heartbreaks started around kindergarten. The boy-crazy phase is very normal for growing girls and childhood crushes are typical, so we weren't abnormal for our boy-craziness. However, we went about it in a very enigmatic and under-the-radar way. We spent a lot of time daydreaming about boys we liked and constantly obsessed over seeing them, being in the same space with them, sharing conversations with them, and getting positive attention from them.

Like we said, we weren't abnormal for liking boys so much, we just experienced high volumes of unnecessary obsessions and experiencing cutting heartbreaks if we didn't get our hearts' desires. In a sense, we didn't have realistic or proportionate crushes. We over-indulged and over-consumed everything about these boys to the point of making us sick. That's what bingeing is—it is over-consuming and feeling stuffed or uncomfortable afterwards.

There were more than a few incidences when we liked a boy and began discussing him and sharing all the wonderful things that we liked about him to the point of feeling nauseous. We obsessed to the point of anxiety and restlessness. We would celebrate at the smallest morsel of attention we would get from these boys that would send us skyrocketing to the moon, but if we felt any sense of rejection, our rockets would come crashing back down to earth.

We can't count how many times we experienced this kind of rejection from our boy-craziness. It wasn't rejection from having mutual feelings with a boy and then finding out they just wanted to be friends with us— No the relationships started in our heads and ended in our heads. Nevertheless, the rejection was real in our hearts.

This cycle went from early childhood all the way into early adulthood—secretly liking boys, mentally dating them, experiencing real life rejection, getting our hearts broken, and then moving on to the next boy crush. It was a different kind of boy-bingeing. We binged on the fantasies of being with them, we binged on replays of interactions with them, imagining being accepted and liked by them. Key words—accepted and liked! That's all we wanted was to be accepted and liked by a boy!

We binged so much secretly, that we became overstuffed—overstuffed with emptiness and hollowness. Bingeing also can include a tendency to "swallow things whole", which Bradshaw describes as a gullible, naïve or passive response in relationships. When you swallow things whole you don't fully chew it and you could choke.[6] You take people as they are and don't challenge people or the things they say. It is such a state of starvation for love that a person misses opportunities to dissect information, spit out what is harmful and keep what is good. Bingeing on boys can definitely make a girl sick!

"IT'S NOT ON THE MENU": FACING REJECTION & HEARTBREAK

Ever go to a restaurant and ask the server if you can have something that is not on the menu? Have you ever gone to Burger King and asked for a "Sizzling Chicken and Cheese" entree? Typically, when you go to a restaurant, you are expected to eat from the selection of what is already provided on the menu. And in most cases, the items on the menu should represent what the restaurant specializes in preparing. So, imagine how baffled the server would be if you asked him/her for something the restaurant does not specialize in making? Furthermore, what might be your motive for even making such an absurd request? Hunger perhaps?

Well, this is how we ended up with so many scars of rejection—we repeatedly found ourselves in situations where we asked guys for stuff they could not give us. We wanted love, acceptance, commitment, fidelity, exclusivity, adoration, affirmation, and loyalty—but were constantly told, "It's not on the menu!" We were constantly sent away just as hungry as we were when we started the connection. One too many times we were left feeling like we were not good enough to get our needs met in relationships. Why? Because we were going to the wrong places to get what we needed. We expected to get something that was unreasonable for the person to give us. We wanted a Sizzling Chicken and Cheese entrée from Burger King.

One of our definitions of rejection is: "the negative emotional consequence as a result of wanting more from a person than they are equipped to give."

Many times, we felt as if maybe there was something wrong with us because a guy did not "want" us, when that wasn't the full truth. The truth was they only wanted certain parts of us and not all of us. Maybe we just weren't their type. Whatever the reasons were for not choosing us, it ended in us feeling rejected. We were left with a lot of heartbreaks and feelings of being unwanted. When you have a daddy hunger, that hunger manifests in relationships. You are hungry for the things you missed from not having a father, like hugs, compliments, princess-treatment, quality time and love. With fatherlessness, you are so hungry for love that you make habits of going to restaurants and asking for things that are not on the menu in hopes that a miracle can be performed in the kitchen. Miracles like:

- Maybe he can grow to love the same values I hold

- Maybe he will be okay with abstinence

- Maybe I can adjust to the sporadic phone calls

- Maybe he will text/call me tomorrow

- Maybe he will make us official soon

- Maybe he will want to marry me

These "maybes" were just set-ups for heartbreak, because with the exception of a few good guys, rarely any chose to live up to these standards. Hunger is a bad position to date from because even when the guy says, "It's not on the menu", you still make the choice to deal with whatever they can feed you. Sigh. We journaled, we cried, we treasured the bits and pieces that these guys gave us and tried to make it all mean something that it didn't. We deluded ourselves. We take responsibility for our unnecessarily broken hearts. We take responsibility for asking for things that were clearly not available. We take responsibility for blaming the guy for rejecting us when really, they were more upfront than we were willing to accept. We take responsibility for expecting treatment that just wasn't "on the menu."

THE INSATIABLE SEARCH FOR A REPLACEMENT DAD

Our hungry hearts led us on a deliberate journey to forage for fatherly love from perceived qualified male figures. We refer to this foraging as daddy-shopping—a common behavior for those suffering from father hunger. Daddy-shopping is the process of scoping out dad-like men or men who are currently fathers and engaging in curiosity about what it would be like to be their daughter. It also includes behaviors like attention-seeking, affirmation-seeking, and adoration-seeking from them. The objective was to pose like the ideal daughter in hopes that these father-like figures would feed our need. We didn't necessarily need to have them adopt us, but we did look for those occasional morsels of fathering to help us thrive.

Prior to our dad-shopping ritual, we mostly attached to men who fit more of a surrogate brother role and whom we perceived to meet various relational and practical needs. This habit came from our fantasy nature and was not based on reality, as many of these relationships were not healthy. We almost wonder if our minds were confused during our adolescence and early twenties with the misbelief that a big brother would suffice when really what we wanted was a father. Once we started desiring and seeking relationships with father-figures, we didn't entertain all the brotherly relationships much anymore.

There are some great meal replacements out there to offer sustenance and nutrients when a real well-balanced meal isn't available, but the reality is a replacement is still a replacement. Ensure® is great and tasty, but it isn't the same as a salad, fruit, and a chicken wrap for lunch. We loved our temporary father replacement figures, but they couldn't give us everything we needed or be there for us as much as we needed. It is important to radically accept that each person is only due one biological father in this life!

Tish Granville and Lanelle Jackson

CHAPTER 6

THE STARVED SOUL

"What a relief to be empty! Then God can live your life." –Rumi

"The full he empties, and the empty he fills." –Charles Spurgeon

SOUL-STARVATION

Daddy-starvation is one thing! God-starvation is another! To be disconnected from a parent is one thing! To be or to feel disconnected from your Creator is much worse. Our loss of a primary attachment figure and the subsequent starvation led to what felt like a loss of relationship with God at times; a relationship inflicted with depletion, emptiness, and insatiable hunger. Daddy hunger ultimately left our minds malnourished, our hearts hungry and our souls starved. But what exactly do we mean by a "starved soul?"

Well, just like any other living organism that does not have adequate food intake, starvation became the diagnosis for our souls. Our souls basically did not have enough to eat but not because we did not have access to the abundant source of nourishment, it was because we were not sitting down at the table where the provision was. Essentially, we suffered in our ability to maintain our consumption of God when our consumption of the nutrients an earthly father typically provides became a non-reality. We were quite preoccupied with sitting down at a different table— the table where our father should have been serving us all kinds of fatherly delights. We returned day after day to this table where we hoped one day there would be a kind, loving, protective father sitting and inviting us to partake of all that a daughter desires from her father—only to find an empty seat. This table of supposed feasts and broken bread (with butter) became a table of famine and broken hearts. This table represented unmet needs, abandonment, rejection, letdowns, waiting, sadness, and hunger. But all along God was calling us to a much better table—a table of feasts and broken bread (with butter) where we could become filled and blessed. We would never go hungry again because we could come and fill up whenever we wanted—and the seat of our Savior would NEVER be vacant. He would always be there, inviting us to sit and sup with Him.

But we did not make that choice to sit at the table with God enough—which lead to our soul-starvation. Our souls began to lack the nutrients needed to make us into the women of God we were created to be. To have a starved soul is to have a soul that lacks the spiritual nutrients of love, joy, peace, patience, kindness, goodness, faithfulness, gentleness, and self-control—edibles that can only come from sitting at God's table. We will talk more about how God truly filled us with His delicious provisions a bit later, but during this period of soul-starvation, it's important that we share with you how we developed these starved souls from both an interpersonal and a spiritual perspective.

FAILING TO FEAST OUR EYES ON GOD

We know the spiritually correct thing to say is that God is enough and that He alone should satisfy our hearts. We know the faith community often goes bananas if you confess that you want God plus _____ (fill in the blank). But the truth of the matter is that God made us to need Him more than anything else but not necessarily to need Him only. He made us to need relationships. He made babies to need parents, men and women to need spouses, gals and guys to need friends. He made us to have vertical connection (with Him) and horizontal connection (with others). In the garden, He had all the goodness of Himself to offer to Adam. He could have engaged in an exclusive relationship with Adam, but instead He said, "It is not good for man to be alone." What? Adam was alone even with the presence of God almighty? How could that be? Here we have the establishment of the horizontal relationship. So, to not have the love of a biological father and still feel heartbroken with God in the garden with us is not an indictment on our faith. God made us this way.

While we do recognize that we have this hunger for dad and that it is not going to go away simply because we have God in the garden, we also recognize that God made us to feast on Him and enjoy wholeness through Him in such a way that we will not be consumed by the breakdowns in our horizontal relationships. We know this now—but we did not process this well in our earlier years. We struggled to feast our eyes on God. Our hearts didn't always pitter-patter in the presence of God. We didn't always know to look at Him with expectation that He would comfort us in our hunger pain. And because we didn't see all the goodness of scooting our chairs up to the Divine Table, we missed out on a lot of His soul-healing and soul-filling banquets. And when we did sit and dine, we would often eat and run. You know, when you don't really want to engage with those at the dinner table so you sit only for the purpose of getting your grub on, and then after you take that last bite, you take off? So rude right? Dinner is not about the food as much as it is about the communion, the conversations, the contact, the connection, and the comfort. To leave dinner prematurely (after you stuffed your face), is sometimes a message of, "I don't want you, just your food." And that's no way to treat the Heavenly Father (or our loved ones). Yet we failed to feast more times than we care to admit.

Parents set the Table

Human relationships are very powerful. They have the power to hurt us in ways we cannot even fathom and benefit us in ways that our hearts cannot contain. A mother and father possess great power over their child, even to the point of influencing the development of a faulty narrative of God.

One model of parent-child relationships suggests that children view God through the example set by their parents—or through the table set by their parents. This means that initially, children do not have a clear God-concept. This concept develops with age. Early on, a child's most concrete and tangible representation of God is their mother and father. Remember, children are very concrete, they cannot think abstractly until adolescence, and much of spirituality is nontangible and abstract. It is the mother and father who help the child develop a sense of who God is through the behaviors, emotions, and attitudes they respond to the child with. The parent must essentially set a table that prepares the child to eventually sup with God. How the parent treats their vulnerable child can be misinterpreted by the child as treatment they should expect to receive from God. A parent's presence or absence is often assumed to represent either the presence or absence of God in the child's life. A child makes the assumption, "If mom/dad is this way, God must be this way too!"

We attribute our soul-starvation to this model. We had an absent father and sometimes physically and emotionally absent mother, so we developed a soft-core belief that God was absent too. We had to make sense of who God was through our brokenness and through an unset table. We did not know what it was to be protected, be affirmed, be loved, or even be known by a father. And additionally, we do not "know" our father, we do not know his character and what he looks like, we did not get to see his strength or benefit from his provision and protection. So how could we feel these things from God? How could we know God to be these things when we had no father to represent Him? How could we "know" God, His character, His ways and His heart when we had no earthly father as our link and connector?

Our soul-starvation and hunger was defined by our inability to feel known, loved, felt, heard, seen, and touched by God because we were never known, loved, felt, heard, seen, or touched by a father. We struggled for many years to receive God's love and nourishment, because we didn't have a father to set the table. We had a lot of questions about who God was and what He could do:

- Can God protect me?
- Will He affirm me?
- Is He there?
- Is He approachable?
- Does He love me?
- Will He show up?
- Can He meet my needs?

And these questions left us hungry—because we were answering these questions based on how we answered them regarding our father—big, enormous NO'S! How did your caretakers set the table for you?

"Let the Children Come to Me"

We do not believe it was God's intention for human relationships to have that much power over us either way—to be constant sources of rejection or addiction. And we do not believe God intended for His creation to relate to Him through the filters of pain and hurt accrued from human relationships, yet here we are trying to sort it all out.

Scripture does not say a lot about how children view God and specifically the role that parents play, but there is an exceptional story in the New Testament where some parents are trying to bring their children to Jesus and the disciples opposed this, which prompted a rebuke from Jesus. Let's take a peek.

[13] "One day some parents brought their children to Jesus so he could lay his hands on them and pray for them. But the disciples scolded the parents for bothering him. [14] But Jesus said, 'Let the children come to me. Don't stop them! For the Kingdom of Heaven belongs to those who are like these children.' [15] And He placed his hands on their heads and blessed them before he left." (Matthew 19:13-15 NLT)

This text shows two choices that an adult or parent can make in their child's life so that they may not later suffer from soul-starvation: ***Present or Prevent***. A parent can ***present*** their children to Jesus or ***prevent*** them from getting to Jesus. Presenting your children to Jesus goes beyond telling them about Jesus or taking them to church; how you treat your children is also how you present them to Jesus. Preventing your children from coming to Jesus is not limited to not talking about Him or exposing them to His truth; a parent can stop their child from getting to Jesus by being emotionally absent, failing to meet their child's love language, or being abusive and neglectful.

Jesus doesn't want anything to get in the way of children getting to Him. Presenting your children to Him means setting the table up with cutlery, plates, napkins, a tablecloth, a flower vase in the middle and a salt and peppershaker. In other words: attuning to your child, holding their emotions, consoling them, being truthful with them, being kind to them, giving them structure without shaming who they are, disciplining them without destroying them. It means giving them your presence! Did your parents present or prevent?

FORSAKEN AND BEGGING BREAD

God, how could you do this to us? Where were you and where are you now? How are you going to make any good come out of this? Why would you leave us like this? Why aren't you doing anything about this? Why me? Why? Why? Why? —Have you ever asked God these questions? We certainly have. We've wondered where He was and what He was doing and sometimes what He was NOT doing. These are often the sentiments of those who feel forsaken.

To be forsaken is to be ditched, abandoned, left, and deserted. To be abandoned and rejected are easily two of the top 10 worst human experiences—and that is what we felt, not just by our earthly father, but by our Heavenly Father as well. It felt like our prayers were ricocheting off the ceiling. It was as if we were writing letters to God for years and He had the pile of unopened letters on his desk collecting dust. And yet we kept attempting more letters, "Hey, it's me again…I'm not sure if you received the last prayer I mailed off to you, but uh, can you please help?"

With every seemingly unanswered prayer, more confusion and blame began to set in. "Maybe this is all God's fault!"—is the thought that began to creep into our hearts. We began to believe at points in our lives that this was all His doing. We found Him to be guilty of withholding a father from us, which left us hungry for the love of a father.

Of course, we blamed other individuals as well. But we couldn't really blame our father because we weren't sure if he even knew we existed. We held blame towards our mother but began to try and find healing and have worked to release her from our crossfires of blame. So, there is God left— and of course Satan, but ultimately, we reasoned that the All-Powerful God could have intervened and that He was at-fault for us being forsaken and begging for bread.

Have you ever played the blame game? It's not quite as fun as UNO or Connect 4 but many of us have participated in a round or two of it. In this game, you have to find someone to be at-fault for something that has gone wrong in your life. Negative circumstances are not a coincidence nor are they happenstance. Someone or something is to blame for everything that is unpleasant in your story. So, in this game, the objective is to find who or what is to blame and direct your anger, annoyance, attitude and accusations to that thing or person. Also, it is important to mention, that there are no winners in this game. There are no blessings or benefits from blame. And actually it's no fun in it at all—blame is not a game. It will ruin relationships, rupture hearts, ransack connections and rob you of peace and optimal mental health.

Scripture says in Psalm 37:25 (NLT): *"Once I was young, and now I am old. Yet I have never seen the godly abandoned or their children begging for bread."* There are two key promises here to point out: 1) the godly will not be abandoned 2) descendants of the godly will not have to beg for bread (their needs). Our blame of God was tied to our feeling of abandonment. We accused Him because we felt forsaken in our fatherlessness. We spent a lot of time begging for love, affection, connection, protection, nurture and care so we did not feel like this promise applied to us.

How do you cope with the written story of your life that has chapters that you didn't get to approve, amend, or alter before it was published? How do you argue your case with both the author and the supposed hero of the story? How do you reconcile the truth that God promised to never forsake us with the feeling of being forsaken?

No one should ever continuously entertain the unproductiveness that blaming brings. It simply is not helpful. It wasn't helpful to us and brought us no real answers or comfort. We have concluded that God's part in the whole matter has been nothing more than to offer us His sovereignty and grace as we navigated and continue to plunge through life fatherless.

Tish Granville and Lanelle Jackson

CHAPTER 7

THE IDENTITY DEFICIT

"The wounded inner child contaminates intimacy in relationships because he has no sense of his authentic self." –John Bradshaw

"If your daughter doesn't get healthy physical affection from her father while growing up, she will eventually seek that masculine affection she craves from other sources—usually ones you don't want giving her physical affection." -Rick Johnson

God made us to crave Him and become filled up with everything that He says we are. He made us to find our worth, value and identity in Him and Him alone, but somehow, we have adopted an identity based on confusion, emptiness, and hunger for the wrong things. We are craving-beings; however, we crave less of our Creator and more of created things, people, and places. We can be described with many adjectives, but rarely the adjectives God divinely ascribed to us—this is an identity crisis.

We are hungry to know who we are but not hungry enough for the One who can accurately tell us the answer to our questions. These are not good conditions to start a family with. When we are empty of the truth of who we are and we start a family based on this emptiness, we spread our hollowness into our family therefore creating a Family Identity Crisis.

A family identity crisis is a family that has a faulty perception of who it is as a system. A family without an identity is highly dysfunctional, chaotic, broken, distressed, and empty of purpose. The family-system crisis features a.) members that don't know their roles, b.) a home with vacancies in roles, and c.) perversions in roles. It is critical that members within the family know their roles, stay committed to and refuse to abandon their roles, and avoid warping, distorting, and abusing their roles.

If identity does not become secure over time, a transgenerational effect can take place where the identity of the family becomes corrupt for many generations. Yikes! Have you ever done a family genogram? If you have, you may have been able to identify the transgenerational crises in your own family and you can see that patterns can work their way through the bloodline if someone in the family doesn't command the direction of the family.

So how does a family reclaim its identity? To fix the whole, you have to fix the parts. It's imperative that each adult family member address his or her individual identity crisis first.

Here are a few truths about individual identity:

- The foundation of who *I* am is connected to my faith in who God is.

- God is the only one who can fill *my* life and satisfy *my* hunger.

- *I* am God's workmanship (which in the Greek means Poiema or His poem) It takes time to write a poem and each word is chosen carefully and intentionally.

- *My* identity is not "who" *I* am but "whose" *I* am. *I* belong to God.

- *My* identity doesn't change because of where *I* am and who *I* am around. What God says about *me* never changes.

- There is only one of *me*. So *I* better get going being the best me *I* can be.

- *My* identity is not based on what has happened to *me* or *my* ancestors.

- Insert your own truth here: "*I* am _____!"

Now let's translate these truths to define family identity:

- The foundation of who *we* are is connected to *our* faith in who God is.

- God is the only one who can fill *our* family and satisfy *our* hunger.

- *We* are God's workmanship.

- *Our* identity is not about who *we* are but about "whose" *we* are. *We* belong to God.

- **Our** family identity doesn't change because of where *we* are and what other families *we* are around.

- There is only one family like *us*. So let's fulfill *our* mission.

- *Our* identity is not based on generational patterns

- Insert your family truth here: "*We* are _____!"

THE ROLE, RESPONSIBILTY AND IDENTITY OF FATHERS

One of the goals of this book, through our pain, is to contribute to the improvement of our family systems and to help families reclaim their identity. This requires members to reclaim their individual identities—so we want to spend more time directly helping men and fathers in this section. Men you need to know these "UNS."

Unparalleled Role (unrivaled)

Fathers need to know that there is no other role like yours. There is no parallel, no comparison, no replacement, no identical role to who you are in the family. Dads are sort of the GPS unit of the family. As dad goes, so goes the family.[1] We would argue that many fathers have abandoned their role because they are not convinced that they are truly unique, especially in homes of people of color. Men have been beaten down, degraded, dogged, discouraged, and demonized to the point where they believe the role of fatherhood is too big for them to manage, so someone else can do it. Well, no one else can do it…no one can father the child you conceived better than you can. The more that men begin to engrave upon their hearts that they have an unparalleled role as a father, the more they can stand up in their role with confidence, courage, capability, and Christlikeness. If you are a father reading this—let this sink into your heart. Your role matters! You matter! Your family needs you! Your child needs you! The community needs you! The world needs you! God called you! God equipped you! Your child(ren) is/are a gift! Your role as a father is the best role in the world! Occupy it!

Undeniable Responsibility

Well, every role has responsibilities. For example, if you are a secretary (your role), then you will most likely be answering phones, faxing, emailing, filing, sorting, and managing various other administrative tasks (your responsibilities). When the secretary calls off sick, someone else must figure out how to execute those duties. Chances are that a fill-in may not administrate quite like the secretary. Their presence will be missed and the team around them will be anxious for their return.

Similarly, a father has undeniable responsibilities. When he vacates his role, someone else must figure out how to execute his tasks—and the truth is—no one else can. Others can try to do their very best, but it is highly likely the fill-ins are crossing their fingers and hoping "dad" reclaims his responsibilities.

Fathers, you need to understand this—no one can do what you do, the way that you do it! This is an indisputable truth—you are needed, and you are unique in your assignment. To us, there is no other side to the argument. Yes, we understand there are exceptions like death, sickness, mental illness, and divorce that necessitate another loved one taking on fatherly responsibilities and we are all in favor of this. What is important is that fathers begin to consider heavily, that if it comes down to a choice to abandon your responsibilities, you should never!

Unbreakable Identity

Fathers need to know that their identity is sealed. It is unshakeable— unchangeable—unbreakable! Identity is all about who God says you are which means, whatever He says, is the final say. God called you a father to your children. You are a royal priesthood! You are chosen! You are called! Your mistakes can't change your identity in God! Your history or past can't destroy it—unless you allow it to! Your job status or IQ can't alter it! Your identity is to be a father who is worthy of his calling—a warrior—wonderfully made—and a worshipper! That's right, fathering and taking care of your children is an act of worship. So keep fighting to hold on to these truths and take your place as king.

MOTHERS CAN'T BE FATHERS

Growing up without a father was certainly a blow to our understanding but seeing our mother trying to do both–now that was an even bigger blow to our understanding. While she did the best she could to protect us, provide for us, discipline us, and educate us, she should not have had to.

She was doing more than half of what she was called to do. Even in healthy homes where there is a mother and father, there will be the occasional switching and filling in of roles to keep the home running, but single mothers do not have anyone to delegate those extra roles to. It's just them---doing everything! They unconsciously go about their parenting trying to give their children everything that they think they need, not knowing that all their pouring out can still leave the child feeling empty.

Back to our mother, she had to work, cook, clean, educate and help us with homework, get her own education, have her own social life, discipline us, drive us places, provide for us a home and safe environment, and so much more. In all her doing, we still needed so much more. We taught ourselves how to ride bikes. We did not always have that affirmation. We had to teach ourselves how to conduct relationships with the opposite sex.

There is just no way she could teach us everything and give us all the nutrients we needed. Like any other single mother, stepping in and out of the father role can be both exhausting and non-productive. We are proud and honor everything our mother did and what other single mothers do for their kids. Even the mothers who have uninvolved fathers in the home, we commend the efforts and are in awe of the mothers who fight for their kids.

While this is not an easy position to be in for mothers, the truth remains that God never meant for mothers to be alone. He never meant for mothers to have to raise their kids without the input, support, and partnership of a father. The mother and father are supposed to be the support beams that hold a family together. With only one support beam, the whole system is at risk of collapsing and crumbling.

Fathers are supposed to be there to hold mom up when she becomes mentally and physically weak from parenting and vice versa. We already provided the specific nutrients that fathers offer in chapter 3 so imagine a mother having to do her part and someone else's. It's not impossible, but it is hard to try and offer all those nutrients to one or more children. A single mother could provide 5 nutrients one day, the next day 7, the next day 3, and the next day 10, but she can never provide all of them. Even with two healthy parents, the ball can drop, but that margin of error dramatically increases with a single mom.

When mothers are willingly or circumstantially put in a position to parent their children alone, they are left with the difficult task of trying to provide all the necessary nutrients that children need to thrive. Since this task is daunting and just not possible, mothers are left worn out and children are left neglected and unattended to in various areas. Children don't experience the balanced parenting with a free flowing of nutrients that help them to thrive and stay emotionally healthy. They miss out on so much which is where the malnutrition and underdevelopment comes into play.

Again, we salute every mother who did it alone or who is currently doing it alone. We can only encourage you and pray strength for your journey. We do not minimize your experience, but we do maximize the hope that although you may feel alone, a community of like-minded women stand with you. And for the children, like us, who are a result of single mothering, there is hope for you too. Missing fathers have created an enormous hole in families, but we have the responsibility to recognize the intended purpose of fathers and to use our pain and hurt to propel forward and begin building stronger families and communities from now on.

HUSBANDS *SHOULDN'T* FATHER THEIR WIVES

The desperation for a father has no end it seems. For us, relationships with boys didn't pan out. Big brothers came and went. Father-figures had expiration dates—but there was still one more option—get married and have our father hunger needs fulfilled by our husbands—or so we thought. We can't deny the fact that we entertained the idea of our husbands putting our daddy-pain to rest for good. The idea may not have been a fully conscious thought, but it was certainly subliminal. We thought there was a chance our hearts could be healed inside of the context of marriage if our husbands played "daddy" occasionally. We thought marriage was some sort of package deal or restitution plan provided by God—until we came to grips with the reality—Husbands shouldn't be fathers to their wives.

Marriage provides a safe place and can be a sacred setting to receive an abundance of healing and heart-help for fatherless adults, male or female, but a spouse is not a replacement for an absent parent. Marriage was not the place for us to receive our replacement dad. It was critical that we recognized this very early on. We are both very cognizant of how our father wounds can become triggered in marriage and we did our best not to project onto our husbands, but we can't confirm that there haven't been times where our spouses were not put on the father pedestal.

Understanding your role within the family is important. The overall identity of the family is dependent on its members knowing and fulfilling their appropriate roles. We do not expect this to be a widely agreed upon objection but based on our understanding of how family systems work best, we do not believe husbands should try to fill the shoes of an absentee father for their wives. It is a conflict of interest. It's a dual-relationship that can complicate the health of the marriage.

4 Key reasons why husbands should not try to be a father to their wives.

1. God Made Marriage to be Interdependent

God designed marriage to be between a man and his wife; two adults—body, mind, and spirit. God did not design marriage to be between a man and the child living inside of the wife who is subconsciously marrying her idealized father. Marriages that function based on a.) a woman who uses her husband to be her father and b.) a husband who parents and fathers his wife, are dependent and co-dependent relationships. In this case, the wife functions as the dependent and the husband functions as the co-dependent. So, we are all on the same page, our definition of dependent is putting your capabilities off on someone else and co-dependency is enabling someone and preventing them from exercising their capabilities.

In childhood, parents are supposed to foster dependency within the child as the child cannot meet their most significant needs. If the child does not have reliable parents or has absent parents, the child grows up with unmet needs and eventually becomes an adult who may be overly dependent or under-dependent on others. A woman who grows up without learning healthy dependence may have two versions of herself, the competent version and the dependent version. She is fully capable in many ways but when her daddy hunger begins to inconvenience her, she becomes dependent in areas where her adult-self is pretty capable. The husband then has a choice; to enable her or help her to grow herself up in a healthy way.

A woman who seeks to have a father in her husband creates a cycle of dependency on him to do things for her that she can do for herself—this contradicts a healthier model of marriage that typifies interdependence. Interdependence is a synergy between husband and wife where they both balance the art of leaning on and supporting each other—it is a mutual reliance on one another.

2. The Husband Endures Periods of Wifelessness

During the time that a woman is reenacting her child-like needs from the past, her husband is temporarily without a wife. Let us say that again—when a wife regresses and needs her husband to be her father, this means he is without a wife during those episodes. If he has any adult needs during these regressions, he faces the reality of having them go unfulfilled due to his wife's unavailability.

If the wife sees him as her father in overt or covert ways this forces him out of his role as husband, particularly if he is not perceptive enough to stay grounded in his role. He switches from having a wife to having a daughter that looks very much like his wife and sounds very much like his wife, but isn't quite his wife. He may scratch his head with confusion and try to approach it logically and if all else fails he has to retreat and wait for his wife to come back to the present—leaving him without his companion for that time. He may go to the gym, go for a drive, go into his man-cave, go to bed early, go hang with some friends, or escape into the tv until his wife returns from her voyage back to childhood.

3. The Wife Develops Unhealthy Expectations

A wife who regresses into states of a little girl needing her daddy may inappropriately raise her expectations of her husband. She expects things of him that are outside of his boundaries as her husband. He may be a praiseworthy mate; doing his very best to meet her needs—she may even feel fulfilled being his wife, but when she slides out of her role as wife, she overlooks his performance as her husband and begins to question if he is meeting her needs or not.

She will demand more. She will expect more—not realizing it is her little girl crying out for more within her. A wife who expects her husband to be her father will place pressure on him to do double duty. In an unspoken protest she may demand, "After you are done tending to me, I need you to tend to the little girl within me." If the husband does not meet her expectations to satisfy both her adult needs and her child-based needs, she will become very unhappy and protest even more.

Here are some more potential expectations of a wife who needs her husband to be her father:

- make decisions for her that she should be empowered to make for herself

- discipline her and "train" her

- give her excessive attention and affection outside of the boundaries of a sacred marriage

- rescue her from her emotions

- protect her from challenges that she needs to experience

- be responsible for her improved self-esteem

- care for her in ways she should be able to care for herself

- avoid hurting her or ever breaking her heart

4.) The Marriage Lacks Reciprocity and Balance

When a woman regresses to her younger self, she starts to see her husband as her father and therefore needs fatherly nutrients from him. She may be very fulfilled as a wife but when she becomes triggered; her emptiness begins to protest for more from her husband. The love that her husband is providing her is much different than the love that she needed from a father. This causes her to feel like she is constantly lacking something and that her poor husband is never doing enough. If the husband cannot tolerate the tension he will submit and play the role of father to keep his wife happy. This puts him in a position of pursuing as a husband and parenting as a father which puts his wife on the receiving end more than the marriage can support.

The husband must do a lot of emotional support and caretaking and he may not be getting the care he needs in return. We understand 50/50 relationships rarely exist, nor are they necessarily indicators of a healthy relationship. In many cases, it is quite normal and functional for a relationship to be 60/40, 70/30 and 80/20 during various seasons of marriage. There are times where mates switch roles in who acts as the pursuer and who acts as the responder and times and experiences where spouses take turns giving and receiving from one another.

Furthermore, God did not design marriage to be tit-for-tat or score-card driven; He designed for it to be sacrifice-driven. Scripture says it is more blessed to give than it is to receive (Acts 20:35, NASB), and we want to be sure our admonition for balance lines up with this truth. If both mates hold the same value that they have great capacity and intention to give, then the marriage will naturally stay in balance—both mates will give sacrificially to one another. When a wife needs her husband to father her, she is neglecting her call to give, and this puts the marital balance at risk. Mate-to-mate reciprocity is lost and replaced with a parent-to-child system of relating.

The Culture Effect

The culture and times that we live in have their own influence on the matter of if a husband should be a father to his wife when needed. There are always two sides to every argument. We want you to be well informed of both arguments and the suggestions from the culture that support the dual role a husband can play for his fatherless wife.

The culture posits these pros for Husband/Father roles:

- The wife can get the healing that she needs in a safe relationship
- The husband is the most available male in her life so why not?
- It won't hurt anyone
- It's a sign of his true love for her
- It's his duty to help her
- It's many women's dream to have a husband who "fathers"
- He will only have to do it temporarily

These positions seem so anodyne and without consequence and are even addressed in mainstream music. Check out these modified lyrics from the song "Father in you", by one of Hip-Hop's legendary singers Mary J. Blidge. She sings:

When I was a little girl
I didn't have a father
And that's why
I'm leaning on you
When I was a baby
I didn't get a hug
From daddy that's
Why I need a hug from you
Oh it's not easy
And I thank you for putting up with me
When u don't have a daddy's love
That's why I need the father in you (repeat chorus)
Whoa things got bad to the point where mommy couldn't hold us down
And that's when it hurt me so much to see her (To see her cry)
Oh don't cry mom, don't cry mom
We're gonna be alright
That's what I used to say
That I would try to take his place
(But it was too hard) it was so hard
Trying to be a man not a woman
(And that's why I need the father in you)

There are ad-libs in the song where she really pleads with her husband not to hurt her, not to let her down and to be true to her. At the end of the song, she goes on to encourage other men to be there for their significant others who don't have a father and appeals, "don't ignore her." While no one wishes for hurt in their marriage, it is an expected experience. It is unrealistic to restrict your spouse from hurting you due to father-wounds. She also emphasizes that she needs her husband to hug her because her father neglected to do so. Affection is a normal and healthy need within marriage, and we can see the significance of her need for more hugs in her marriage because of her childhood. As you can see, the idea of a husband fulfilling his wife's deficits from fatherless is normalized in her expressions.

This song really highlighted a topic that is not often expressed in music culture, and it has some validity to it. While we do not believe a husband should play a father-role to his wife, we do believe there are some qualities that he can provide that can be very healing and appropriate for her.

Husband as Haven

It's important that we validate the husband in his role and lay out some healthy expectations a wife can have. There are many healthy and functional ways for a marriage to be a haven for women who grew up fatherless or with father wounds without compromising the sacredness of the marriage. It can be done, so please be encouraged.

There is some over-lap in what fathers and husbands provide, so this can be very useful for those with deficits emotionally and relationally.

Fathers and husbands both provide:

- Protection- It is not uncommon for a woman to look for her husband to keep her protected and safe just as a father would do. A husband can stand up for his wife when she is being targeted, he can defend her against others who wrong her, he can lock doors and call and check on her when he is away from her, he can make sure she has made it to her destination when she travels and commutes alone. There is no limit to the way a husband can cover and look after his wife. If these basic needs of protection are being met, then it is likely that a woman with father wounds will find healing in the marriage.

- Affection- Most women have a primary need for affection. This can include hugs, kisses, cuddling, terms of endearment, a warm smile, and other physical and verbal gestures of love. These are also gestures that a loving father provides. In most instances, the best type of affection is the kind the wife doesn't have to ask for. This provides a type of security that she needs to feel loved within the marriage. A woman with father wounds may have a magnified need for affection and it can be healthy for her to recognize when she needs affection and to ask for it in a healthy way. The key is that when affection is provided, she gives herself permission to heal and grow herself back up. It can also be helpful to say, "Thank you, I really needed that" when affection is initiated during a time where she needed it the most.

- Financial support- In most family contexts, a father has a role of providing financial support voluntarily for his family and children. This should not have to be asked of him in a healthy context; it is already his value and belief system to do so. He does not like to see his children lack anything, whether that is food, clothes, housing, school supplies, diapers, and anything relevant for everyday survival. This is also a quality found in healthy marriages. Most husbands do not like to see their wives lack anything. A husband who takes care of bills and debts, funds groceries for the house, pays for the car to get repaired, and when the furnace goes out, he is on the ball looking for a solution, provides a special type of security for his wife. Even if she contributes financially to the house in an equal or greater fashion, she still relies on the competence in her husband to support her. A woman with father wounds can find healing in a relationship where there is financial support because it can convey the message to her that, she is worthy of being taken care of. If a husband is not able to provide like he would like, that is understandable to her if he continues to affirm her in his desire to do so if he could.

- Leadership-A woman who grew up fatherless may have an innate need for male authority in her life. She may desire guidance, direction, and leadership in order to feel more secure. This is not an uncommon role for husbands to play in marriage. Christian principles on marriage are often based on husbands being the head of the household, not in a tyrannical way but in a loving and trustworthy way. This could mean that husbands are responsible for the vision and mission for the family and outlining the path to get the family to their destination. This could mean making calls, sending emails, making appointments, problem solving, and taking responsibility for errors and decisions. And what about sleepless nights thinking about family goals while the wife and kids are fast asleep? Yes, that too. This does not mean that woman cannot co-pilot or co-lead, it often just means that husbands are in the pilot seat. So, leadership is important for a woman with father wounds; and she can heal within the context of marriage if she shows gratitude for her husband when he makes small or great decisions, takes initiative with family business, and owns his errors as a leader. Women with father wounds should be careful not to idealize or allow tyrant behavior, abuse, control, and co-dependency as this causes re-victimization and delays healing.

The husband can indeed provide a haven for his wife with a history of fatherlessness if he exercises the above qualities inside of healthy marriage boundaries. Whatever he provides for his wounded and recovering wife, he should do with a "Husband-Only" mentality—hug her as a husband, provide for her as a husband, lead her as a husband, and protect her as a husband.

Message to fatherless ladies

If you are still single, begin to look for healthy ways to get your inner-child needs met so that when or if you stand at the altar on your wedding day, you don't have an inappropriate belief that you are getting a two-for-one deal. We don't want you to believe that you are getting a "husband and daddy" all in one as you say "I Do" in front of family and friends. We want you to be free to love your husband and receive love from him from your adult version and allow him to be the husband God has crafted for him to be for you.

Seek out a qualified counselor or spiritual mentor to help you identity the ways in which you may be tempted to use your future spouse to meet your daddy-needs. Read literature and self-help books on your problem-areas. Find a support groups in your community. Go into marriage fully aware of your deficits and get familiar with your protest behavior when your needs are not met.

When you feel comfortable and prepared, let eligible prospects know a little about your story upfront so they can mentally prepare for the challenges and expectations. Come up with a plan for how you will be alerted to your regressions and a plan to grow yourself back up.

If you are married, assess your approach to marriage. Are you aware of episodes where you switch roles and demand things of your husband that only a father could fulfill for you? Do you show gratitude for the protection, provision, affection, and leadership that your husband provides for you? Do you give yourself permission to heal when your husband is meeting your needs, or do you throw a pity party for what your "little girl" didn't get from her father?

Study your behavior and ask for feedback from your mate. You will never be a little girl again and you can never get what your daddy didn't give you from your husband, so the most your husband will be able to do for you in the present is give you feedback and help you brainstorm healthy ways to heal. Remember, much of your healing journey will happen individually—code word for alone! Don't be afraid of that word. But the good news is there are so many parts of your journey where you can have the wonderful company of your spouse. Your husband shouldn't be your father, but he can be your biggest supporter, your coach, your confidant, your reflective mirror, your sounding board, your shoulder to cry on, and your haven.

Message to men married to father-wounded ladies

Take a deep breath! Whatever pressure you have placed on yourself to try to make up for what your wife didn't get in her childhood, adolescence, and young adulthood can now be released. You don't have to be more than her husband anymore. Pat yourself on the back for how you have courageously loved her up to this point while also taking time to reflect on growth opportunities.

Are there areas where you can grow in as a husband? Sure, there are! There are always areas where we can stretch and challenge ourselves but growing in your ability to rid her of her father wounds is not necessarily one of the ways you need to challenge yourself. What you can do is own up to ways you have hurt her or made "matters worse." Own up to ways you have carelessly approached husband-hood or failed to keep your vows. Apologize when you are aware of times you withhold love and affection from her. Assess times where you hit below the belt, push her buttons, and behave in ways that you know are definite triggers. Her regressions are not completely your fault but there may be missed opportunities of consideration that you can monitor.

There is a difference between walking on eggshells and walking with consideration. Scripture says in 1 Peter 3:7, *"Husbands, in the same way be considerate as you live with your wives and treat them with respect as the weaker partner and as heirs with you of the gracious gift of life, so that nothing will hinder your prayers."* If raising your voice scares her, then be considerate of that. If you know she needs hugs, don't skip months before giving her one. Be considerate of her need for affection. Yes, she is responsible for growing herself up, but this does not give license to others to trip her, so she falls down into the pit of regression.

Break free from unhealthy patterns you have allowed to become the norm in your marriage. Are there things you know your wife can do but you enable her instead of pushing her to be her best? Do you allow yourself to feel guilty for her inappropriate expectations of you? Do you boss her around? Do you talk to her like she is a little girl even if that is her subconscious need sometimes? What house chores or family responsibilities can you manage once a week so she can have space to be alone and grow herself back up? If she is too bogged down taking care of the house, children, and your needs, she will inevitably neglect herself (because that's just what women do). If she neglects herself, she will probably regress more. A self-care break once a week will be good for everybody.

Tish Granville and Lanelle Jackson

CHAPTER 8

THE SACRED TABLE

"Look! I stand at the door and knock. If you hear my voice and open the door, I will come in, and we will share a meal together as friends." –Revelation 3:20 (NLT)

Imagine being so hungry that you find yourself staring into a trashcan. Sticky wrappers, ketchup packets, half-eaten sandwiches, wads of paper, and used cups abound. You start rummaging through looking for something to drive the hunger pangs away. At this point, you aren't considering contamination, you just want to end the devastation of starvation. It is clear, deficits drive us to dirty places, destruction, desperation and even into depravity.

Did you know we are more likely to sin when we are hungry? Hunger makes us more vulnerable to temptation—and not just hunger for food—but any hunger that derives from our flesh nature whether that be hunger for people, things, success, money, popularity, power, or sex. Jesus' wilderness experience teaches us this. Most of us would get into all kinds of trouble just off 3 days with no food, let alone 40. But we now have a model for how to handle our hunger—we can turn to Abba—we can turn to His word and be fed by every word He has ever said. When we turn to Him instead of what our flesh dangles in front of us, He deploys angels to meet our greatest needs. So, what dirty places have you found yourself in looking to fill valid needs? And what kind of sin has your hunger led you to? No matter how you answered, you are not alone. And it is time for an upgrade—let's invite the healer of our hearts over for dinner—a meal with Abba at a *Sacred Table for Two.*

Most of us want to know who we are inviting in for this sacred meal. So, let's formally introduce you to your dinner guest and tell you a little about Him. Who is Abba? The word Abba, which is an Aramaic word, is translated to "daddy." We, who are born-again believers and who follow Christ are referred to as the children of God—which makes Him our Father.

John 1: 12-13 (KJV) states: *"But as many as received Him, to them He gave the right to become children of God, even to those who believe in His name, who were born, not of blood nor of the will of the flesh nor of the will of man, but of God."*

This means that we, as His Beloved children, have a right to call Him Abba and rely on the goodness of His fathership. We are joint heirs with Him and never have to believe the lie that we are fatherless again. Now we call Him *"Abba Father." For His Spirit joins with our spirit to affirm that we are God's children.* Romans 8:15, 16 (CEV).

FATHERLY ATTRIBUTES OF ABBA
Love

> *"For God so loved the world (that includes us) that He gave His one and only Son, that whoever believes in Him shall not perish but have eternal life." (Emphasis Added.) (John 3:16 NIV)*

> *"The steadfast love of the Lord never ceases; His mercies never come to an end; they are new every morning; great is your faithfulness." (Lamentations 3:22-23 ESV)*

> *"See what great love the Father has lavished on us, that we should be called children of God! And that is that we are! The reason the world does not know us is that it did not know him." (1 John 3:1 NIV)*

Compassion

> *"As a father shows compassion to his children, so the Lord shows compassion to those who fear Him." (Psalm 103:13 NIV)*

"He heals the brokenhearted and binds up their wounds." (Psalm 147:3 NIV)

"The Lord is gracious and compassionate, slow to anger and rich in love." (Psalm 145:8 NIV)

"Because of The Lord's great love we are not consumed, for his compassions never fail." (Lamentations 3:22 NIV)

Discipline

"For the Lord disciplines the one he loves and chastises every son whom he receives." (Hebrews 12:6-7 ESV)

"For whom the Lord loves He reproves, even as a father corrects the son in whom he delights." (Proverbs 3:12 NASB)

Mercy

"Surely goodness and mercy shall follow me all the days of my life and I will dwell in the house of the Lord forever." (Psalm 23:6 KJV)

"But because of his great love for us, God, who is rich in mercy, made us alive with Christ even when we were dead in transgressions-it is by grace you have been saved." (Ephesians 2:4-5 NIV)

Affirmation

"But to all who have received him, those who believe in his name, he has given the right to become God's children." (John 1:12 ESV)

"I no longer call you slaves, because the slave does not understand what his master is doing. But I have called you friends, because I have revealed to you everything I heard from my Father." (John 15:15 NET)

"For he chose us in Christ before the foundation of the world that we may be holy and unblemished in his sight in love." (Ephesians 1:4 NET)

"For we are his workmanship, having been created in Christ Jesus for good works that God prepared beforehand so we may do them." (Ephesians 2:10 NET)

"–We know, brothers and sisters loved by God, he has chosen you…" (1 Thessalonians 1:4 NET)

Nurturing

"I, even I, am he who comforts you…" (Isaiah 51:12 NASB)

"He will feed his flock like a shepherd. He will carry the lambs in his arms, holding them close to his heart. He will gently lead the mother sheep with their young." (Isaiah 40:11 NLT)

"Though my father and mother forsake me, the LORD will receive me." (Psalm 27:10 NIV)

"…the sovereign Lord will wipe away the tears from all faces…" (Isaiah 25:8 NIV)

"He heals the brokenhearted and binds up their wounds." (Psalm 147:3 NIV)

"Come with me by yourselves to a quiet place and get some rest." (Mark 6:31 NIV)

"As a mother comforts her child, so I will comfort you; and you will be comforted over Jerusalem." (Isaiah 66:13 NIV)

Teacher

"Who is the man who fears the Lord? He will instruct him in the way he should choose." (Psalm 25:12 NASB)

"I will instruct you and teach you in the way which you should go; I will counsel you with My eye upon you." (Psalm 32:8 NASB)

"Thus says the LORD, your Redeemer, The Holy One of Israel: 'I am the LORD your God, Who teaches you to profit, Who leads you by the way you should go.'" (Isaiah 48:17 NKJV)

This sounds like an amazing dinner guest, right? He will not only meet us where we are, but He will come with everything we need to get filled up. All we must do is set the table and wait for Him to knock on the door.

A MEAL WITH ABBA: THE BREAD OF LIFE & THE LIVING WATER

Hungry hearts that crave the love of their daddies don't have to die of starvation. There is a sustaining, satisfying, satiating meal plan consisting of just one liquid and one solid—but not just any liquid or any solid—this meal plan is straight from Heaven! This power-packed but minimal meal can be eaten for breakfast, lunch, dinner and snack in between and has all the nutrients a famished heart needs.

I know it sounds too good to be true, but after 30+ years of famine and trying everything from A-Z and every food group in the relational food pyramid, we found that all we need to heal our hearts completely are two things—the Living Water and the Daily Bread. Ok so we know your next question is "what store sells this and what aisle." "Is this Living Water next to the Dasani?" "Is this Daily Bread next to the Wonder Bread?" Nope. You can't find it in a store. You find it through a Living God—and His name is Jesus.

Boyfriends went stale like week-old grocery store bread. Big brothers turned moldy like the fresh bread you left in the cupboards too long. Father figures had expiration dates that said, "Best if enjoyed by _____" (fill in the blank with the date of your choice). We know all about earthly bread. We know about water that satisfies only for the moment before we were thirsty again. We are very familiar with water bottle labels that promise to be the best water we've ever tasted.

If there is one thing that we have learned through our journey of woundedness, fatherlessness, and heart-hunger, it is that *people are lacking, relationships are often liabilities, and marriage has limitations.* Connection with others to have critical needs met is often a precursor to a let-down. We have learned this the hard way. People are people and were never designed to fill our emptiness. That is a job for Abba. Since God made the heart, He is the only One qualified to heal it and fill it. He knows exactly the kind of nutrition our hearts need to recover from our histories.

Bread of Life

Scripture is chock full of God's promises for hungry hearts. It was God's promises to us that delivered us from a state of being hungry to living full. Here are some of the major insights, blessings, and benefits of partaking of Abba's Bread when weary with daddy hunger:

- **He hears our complaints of hunger**- It's no secret that hunger can bring out the worst in you. It did for us. When a person is extremely hungry, it is common for them to complain and whine. In the Book of Exodus, the children of Israel were so hungry they began to grumble against God and their leaders. They were mad and felt they were being tortured with starvation. Sometimes our prayers for fatherly love came across more like grumbling and complaining too. Sometimes we were mad at God and shook our fists at Him because it felt like we were being tortured and mistreated. And yet God still chooses to respond. It's so comforting to know that even when we don't ask nicely, He is still so loving that He feeds us what we need. While He never rained a father down from heaven in response to our complaining, He gave us something so much better—His love.

  o   Exodus 16:7 (NKJV) - *"and in the morning you will see the glory of the Lord, for He hears your grumblings against Him."*

- **He gives us what we need one day at a time**- Sometimes we want to save up, store up, and hoard what our hearts are hungry for. When something good does happen inter-relationally, it's easy to fear that nothing else good will happen for a while, and so it's best to over-consume from people or experiences. When you are hungry for love, it's commonplace to fear for your future and worry if your needs will be met tomorrow, the next day and the day after that. Our healing required that we learn to depend on God to meet our needs daily. God chose not to lay out an extensive plan for how He would meet our daddy hunger, instead He gave us provisions one day at a time just like he did the children of Israel. He did not want them hoarding bread out of fear. He wanted them to trust Him, therefore He only supplied enough bread from heaven to last for one day at a time.

- o Exodus 16:4 (NASB) - *"Behold I will rain bread from heaven for you; and the people shall go out and gather a day's portion every day..."*

- **No one else can get the credit for filling us**-This is an essential part of recovery—giving the credit to the right person. Boyfriends, big brothers, and father-figures can make many claims in terms of caring for some of our needs. Many of them were instrumental and even necessary. But none of them can dare claim to be *The Bread of Life*. Sometimes we give people too much credit when it comes to satisfying our hearts. We put humans on the thrones of our hearts when that was never the intended place for them. Had there been one person to rescue us from our daddy pain forever, they could have become a forbidden idol. God did not want that. We learned in the Book of John that Jesus had to set the record straight to His followers. He wanted them to be clear that God used Moses to perform many miracles, but it wasn't Moses who provided the bread—it was none other than God the Father. This message is true for us and is true for anyone else who is suffering from a hungry heart. Read the below scripture reference and replace Moses' name with an influential person in your life who you may have given too much credit for filling you up. Remember, healing can happen for you once you give the credit to the right person.

- o John 6:32 (NASB) - *"Truly, truly, I say to you, it is not Moses who has given you the bread out of heaven, but it is My Father who gives you the true bread out of heaven."*

- **He takes what we have and multiplies it** -God performs miracles for hungry people. His Word is all the proof we need.

He cares about our hunger, whether that is hunger for food or hunger for love. He can supply our needs in many miraculous ways, but one very special way is by taking what we already have and multiplying it. If we only have a little bit of the nutrients that fathers provide, God can take that and use it until we have more than we asked for. We've often felt like we were just getting by on scraps. A hug here, a word of affirmation there. A little protection here, a little leadership there. Just scraps. But God doesn't shy away from scraps. He makes a feast once He gets His hands on what we have.

o   John 6:9; 11- v.9 (NASB) - *"There is a lad here who has five barley loaves and two fish, but what are these for so many people?" v.11 "Jesus then took the loaves, and having given thanks, He distributed to those who were seated; likewise, also of the fish as much as they wanted."*

- **Hunger for God above all else guarantees filling**-God cares about our earthly needs, but He desires for us to hunger for Him and righteousness above anything else that we are hungry for, that includes the love of a parent. *We must prioritize our hunger.* When we become so hungry for a father or fatherly love that we ignore our hunger for God, we risk increasing our suffering. God guarantees to satisfy our hunger for Him. That's amazing, because when we are satisfied in God, we tend to be more satisfied with other earthly needs. This does not mean ignoring your hunger for dad. Just take your starvation to God, get hungry for Him, and let Him do His thing! This was a key realization in our healing journey. If you have neglected your hunger for God while in search of fatherly love, take a few steps back and prioritize your hunger.

o   Matthew 5:6 (NIV) - *"Blessed are those who hunger and thirst for righteousness, for they will be filled."*

- **There are temporal and eternal ways to address hunger**- Much of our time has been spent foraging for food to satisfy our hungry hearts—we are not proud of the places we have sought to find fulfillment and we are not proud of the choices of food we have ingested. What we were unaware of at the time was that we were looking for temporary nourishment when we should have been looking for eternal nourishment. There are ways to address hunger that perish, and there are ways that are eternal. If you do any type of grocery shopping at all, you know that there are both perishable and non-perishable food choices to add to your cart. Historically, we have added a lot of perishable items to our carts thinking this was good eating when this was not God's divine grocery list for us. We were never going to gain the full benefits of healing until we stopped gobbling up food that perished, rotted, spoiled, and decayed and started feasting on food that was nonperishable, interminable, life-giving, and eternal. We can go down the list of people and relationships that seemed satisfying but really had expiration dates that determined when they would spoil and go bad. There were people in our lives who were literally only good for a few weeks before the mold started growing. Yuck! No amount of refrigeration, freezing and storage hacks can keep some people around long enough. We learned this lesson over and over. We wish we had read John 6:27 earlier. Daddy hunger can be healed if you pursue the right kind of food—food that endures—and this food only comes from Jesus. He doesn't have an expiration-date sticker on him—He has a seal that guarantees His infinite healing. He never spoils—He gets better and better with each day.

- o John 6:27 (NASB) - *"Do not work for the food which perishes, but for the food that lasts for eternal life, which the Son of Man will give you, for on Him* the Father, God has set His seal."

- **Good things *are* free**- Our culture teaches us that there is nothing free in the world, especially the "good stuff.' We are taught that you must pay premium price for quality goods. 5-star restaurants brag of world-class ingredients and service that will cost you a day's pay to dine. Our culture teaches and promotes that if you want someone to love you, you must give up everything—because the good stuff costs. You must rack up credit cards, give of your time, give your best emotions, and give your body to them as well. We are not taught to reserve our emotional and physical wages and believe we are still fully loveable. We have spent way too much of our emotional, spiritual, and physical wages for things and people who did not satisfy us in efforts to receive love in return. What a waste! What a broken societal system too! God promises we can have what is satisfying, delightful and good and we don't even have to pay for it!

  o   Isaiah 55:2 (NASB) – *"Why do you spend money for what is not bread, and your wages for what does not satisfy? Listen carefully to Me, and eat what is good, and delight yourself in abundance."*

- **Hungry No More**-What a magnanimous claim! It almost sounds too good to be true! When all you know is hunger and someone promises you that you will never have to feel that sensation again—your perfectly plucked eyebrows raise, and you let out a dubious reply of "Really?" Who wouldn't love for hunger to be wiped out and annihilated for good? Who doesn't want the sensation of being filled and satisfied to be the norm? Well, this is what Jesus promises and we all know His word is truth! But there is a criterion—to access the promise, you must access the Lord of the promise. To taste the bread, you must abide with the Bread. The cool thing about Jesus is He is always ready; He's just waiting on partakers. He has always had the solution to our daddy hunger—He's simply been waiting on us to come to Him. No other relationship, nor male can make such a claim to permanently rid us of our heart-hunger, yet so much time was lost expecting man-made bread to do the miraculous. Forehead slap! If you are like us, don't waste another day eating bread that will continue to induce more hunger. Take hold of the promise and abide with the Bread of Life for a hunger-ending experience.

○ John 6:35 (NASB) – *"Jesus said to them, 'I am the bread of life, the one who comes to me will not be hungry...'"*

Living Water

Of course, Abba wouldn't give us such filling and healing bread without something refreshing and restorative to wash it down with. When you are hungry, you are often thirsty as well and Abba has the best water there is to chase down His life-giving bread—The Living Water.

Scripture is also replete with God's promises for the thirsty soul. Here are some of the major insights, blessings, and benefits of partaking of Abba's Living Water to heal from daddy hunger:

- **Pant for God**-Just like the deer, we panted. Our souls panted and desperately needed God. Sometimes we didn't know that's what our souls were thirsty for because there were so many different water brooks that captivated our attention above God. We panted after men, we panted for attention, we panted for love, we panted for father figures, we panted to be number one in some male's life. There is an urban phrase used often to describe desperation in dating and the pursuit of a romantic partner called being "thirsty." If someone describes you as "thirsty" using this vernacular, they are saying you are desperate and not in an attractive way. You are relentless in your attempts to get someone's attention, perhaps a date with them, perhaps their phone number, perhaps a relationship with them. You don't care about embarrassing yourself. You don't care if they turn you down repeatedly. You just want to win them over by any means necessary and often ignore any clues or cues that suggest the person is not interested. While we have never been labeled as thirsty, our actions sometimes were. We are so glad that we learned that there is a man who will never turn us down if we pursue Him; He will never reject us, never ignore our attempts, never dismiss us. His name is Jesus, and He likes when people are thirsty and panting for Him. He gets glory from the desperation. Getting free from daddy hunger requires a desperation for God and panting for Him. If you have a story like ours, we encourage you to obey your thirst—pant after God.

- o   Psalm 42:1-2 (NASB) - *"As the deer pants for the water brooks, so my soul pants for you, O God."*

- **His Passion Heals us**- Jesus is passionate about providing for us. Scripture says he cried out for us to come to Him if we are thirsty. Pause for a moment and imagine the scene in the scripture below: imagine Jesus enjoying a nice meal and then abruptly standing up, pushing his dinner chair back and yelling with tears in His eyes, "Come get your father voids filled with me!" Can you see the passion in His face? Can you hear the emotion and echoing volume in His voice? Can you see his outstretched hands? Is He looking directly at you when He says it? Are you wondering what made Him disrupt dinner to tell you this? Go ahead and engage with this scene. The reason why this scene is so striking to us is because much of our lives we have longed for someone (a male) to passionately say something along those lines to us— "Hey beautiful, let me be everything you need." In today's relationships most people have a long list of needs they want met, but very few people boast about being the one to meet others' needs. In this text, Jesus is making it very clear that He wants to be the one to meet our every need. Now that's love right there. His passion to allow us to drink from Him whenever we want to provide healing for our father wounds.

- o   John 7:37 (NASB) - *"Now on the last day, the great day of the feast, Jesus stood up and cried out, saying, 'If anyone is thirsty, let him come to Me and drink.'"*

- **Our Belief Heals Us**- Living with daddy hunger has a way of drying out the heart. Because we didn't feel we received the nourishment that we needed, it has often felt like we subsequently had nothing to give. There has been a limited outflow of love due to our dry, desert-like hearts. Now, relationship laws suggest that when you aren't receiving enough deposits, you naturally won't have much to withdraw, but spiritual law says something different—by believing in Jesus, the driest of hearts can have something to give. How amazing! Our belief in Jesus will heal our hearts to the point where instead of there being a drought and emptiness and failure to give love to others, we will instead have a river of life flowing out. No matter the wounding, Jesus promises His living water will flow right into those wounded inner parts. Because like water, Jesus goes where we can't.[1] That means God waters those dry, wounded places and turns them into places of life, abundance, and healing that will be a blessing to both you and others.

- o   John 7:38 (NASB) – *"The one who believes in Me, as the Scripture said, 'From his innermost being will flow rivers of living water.'"*

- **Broken Cisterns Compromise Healing**- This insight stings a little but getting healed has meant apologizing for offending God each time we left his water source and created alternative ways to fill our voids for daddy. Trying to get filled up apart from God is a no-no! Silly us for using our cracked, broken, and damaged vessels to try to collect and store sustainable love. No wonder we always ended up feeling let down. Cracked containers can't contain much at all. It's only a matter of time before emptiness ensues again with the use of broken cisterns. It breaks God's heart to see His children getting poured into, only to see it all seep out of the cracks. When we take things into our hands and try to fix ourselves, it is offensive to God and is going to get us nowhere. We can't fix ourselves! It compromises our healing and stalls the recovery from father wounds.

  - o   Jeremiah 2:13 (NASB) - *"For my people have committed two evils: They have abandoned Me, the fountain of living waters, to carve out for themselves cisterns, broken cisterns that do not hold water."*

- **He won't forsake the thirsty-**For every time we've felt poor in heart and needy and tried to get what we needed to no avail and the hunger and thirst grew and grew, Jesus promised to answer our need and to never forsake us. It is outside of His character to see His children thirsty and turn a blind eye and take His water elsewhere. He doesn't make excuses for why He can't quench our thirsts. He doesn't scrutinize our worthiness of taking a drink. What is interesting is, sometimes He is a last resort for the thirsty. He sees us wandering around with our tongues hanging out of our mouths looking for water and coming up empty. He sees us wandering around from person to person, looking for love and looking for fathering and coming up empty. And He knows the people we are seeking out cannot help us. So, He says, "Enough is enough! I will give them the water they need MYSELF!" When others forsake our need for acceptance and love, God steps in and waters every dry place.

  o Isaiah 41:17 (NASB) - *"The afflicted and needy are seeking water, but there is none, and their tongue is parched with thirst; I, the Lord, will answer them Myself, as the God of Israel I will not forsake them."*

- **Put the Water on His tab-** It really hurts when you need something so desperately—like love—and are made to feel as if you must earn it! Human relationships are quite conditional and are qualification oriented. You must have good credit with people to get their heart, their time, and their attention. If you are not qualified, then you will get the worst that they have to offer and must pay higher rates. We've gone broke, gone in debt, and gone bankrupt trying to pay for basic human needs like love, affection, commitment, care, concern, loyalty, worth and value. Some ways we have paid is by being "good", "cooperative", "agreeable", and "compliant" with others. Pause: What ways have you tried to pay for love? Paying for our hearts to be filled was not God's plan for our hearts to be healed. And it's not His plan for any of His children. God has all the basic human needs we could ever want—and they are all free! Without cost! On the house! And to be frank, if it did cost, it should cost triple all the money in the world because of how supernatural it is. Isn't that so amazing—that not only is what God offers free—but it's the best stuff the fatherless could ever hope for!

o Revelation 21:6 (NASB) – *"Then He said to me, 'It is done. I am the Alpha and the Omega, the beginning, and the end. I will give to the one who thirsts from the spring of the water of life without cost.'"*

- **No More Well Water-** The story in John 4 featuring the Woman at the Well is packed with so much for those who have wounded hearts. It's about a woman with some potential relationship wounds and Jesus used her story to reveal to each of us that He cares about our souls, but He also cares about our failing relationships and our quests for connection and fulfillment! In the story, the woman is dependent on well water, but Jesus offers her water that is unfailing and ever flowing. We know what it's like to be dependent on "well water". You know what well water is right? It's the "Well, I like you but....", "Well, you're a nice girl and all but......", "Well, I like hanging with you but......", "Well, you are like daughters to me but.....", "Well, I'd like to mentor you but...." type of people. Well water is failing water! When we encountered Jesus at the place of our "well", He offered us His unfailing water. He doesn't make up excuses about why He can't meet our needs. Another cool highlight of the story is that Jesus confronted the woman's relationship issues. We're totally paraphrasing here, but Jesus basically says, "Hey, I know about all the men." We don't know why she was on guy #6 but we can make assumptions (You must read the story). We can totally relate. We've made some silly mistakes—wait---no, we've sinned against God in our many pursuits for love. We've sipped from pails filled with failing water and Jesus knows about every sip! And He knows about yours too! He called us to ditch our pails and ditch the well and drink from Him.

That includes ditching any vain attempts at getting our father wounds healed too! We never have to be thirsty for people, relationships, love, and validation again. No more well water! **At the end of the story the woman literally leaves the scene excitedly and she forgets her water pot.

- o John 4:14 (NASB) - *"But whoever drinks of the water that I will give him shall never be thirsty; but the water that I will give him will become in him a fountain of water springing up to eternal life."*

- **Thirsty No More**-The ultimate promise for the thirsty fatherless soul is one glorious day, God promises to do away with all hunger and all thirst. But for now, there will be ongoing thirst signals which are useful for avoiding dehydration[2], there will be dehydration, will still be some tears to shed, there will still be sore memories, there will be pain, there will still be temptations to sip from pails of failing water—but it's all temporary. We are in for some tough days ahead as we navigate life without dad, and we will have to constantly rely on Abba and all the nutrients He provides for us. We have been given an abundance of earthly promises for our emptiness and brokenness, but one day we won't have to strive for healing anymore. We won't know what daddy hunger is. We won't know emptiness. We won't know heartbreak. We will forever be full—and we will never cry again. Let this promise resonate for you too—your daddy hunger is only temporary!

- o Revelation 7:16 (NASB) - *"They will no longer hunger nor thirst…"*

LIVING ON FULL

Through all the details of our HERstory, you now have a taste of our experience with fatherlessness through all the stages and phases of our lives. Maybe you even have a fuller understanding of the importance of fathers and their relevance in the lives of their children. You may have never thought about daddy hunger in the way we have so carefully illustrated—we honestly didn't even understand the depths of our own hunger until we began writing these pages. Some of you reading may have even been able to reflect on your own areas of emptiness as it relates to fatherlessness or whatever figure you would fill in the _____lessness blank with. You may have noticed your own heart, soul or mind "growling" with hunger and made aware of your own need for nourishment. With that being said, we aren't done yet. We gave you a peak into the redemptive work of Christ in our lives in this chapter and we won't dare conclude our story about daddy hunger without sharing with you what a life living on full is like. After Jesus gives His bread and His water, your life changes from the inside out—you live full!

What does living on full mean exactly? Let's examine what the symptoms of *living empty* are like first:

- Not having enough

- Difficulty concentrating on relevant tasks due to hunger

- Poor decision making due to malnourishment

- Desperate behavior

- Surrendering to temptations to fill up with unhealthy things

- Complaining about hunger

- Deficiencies in every area of life

- No energy

Living on Full for us is quite the opposite:

- We have enough and even more than enough of everything our hearts had been longing for in the past and we know who our source is when we need to be refilled up again. Fullness means you don't have to consume foolishness anymore. It means you are satisfied.

- We can now concentrate on all the beauty of life like family, career goals, our purpose, our passions, our relationships, and finally we can concentrate on Jesus. No more being distracted with those nagging hunger pangs.

- Our decision-making has improved because we have all the right nutrients when we are full. We have wisdom, truth, and understanding operating in a fuller capacity whereas before, these vitamins were deficient. We have less and less "ooops" experiences on our record the more we grow up in God. We can take more time to think about our actions before we act. These are things we did not do well on "E."

- We have cultivated our desperation for God. Living full means no longer feeling desperate for someone to father us or love us in that deep fatherly way. Yes, we still desire it—but desire and desperation are two different experiences. We better manage our fears that cause us to act unbecomingly, unrighteous, or unattractively to get our needs met.

- When Jesus fasted 40 days, he was no doubt hungry—and that is when he was faced with temptation. Being hungry for love and fathering made us very vulnerable to temptation, but unlike Jesus, we gave in in the past. Living on full means more power to stand up to the temptations to go outside of God's will for love and connection. We are still faced with temptations to indulge in unhealthy fillers, but we have improved in our ability to stay inside of the boundaries God set for us.

- You know a person is hungry because they are often verbalizing how hungry they are every 5 minutes in a no-doubt valid complaint. Praise Jesus the days of complaining every 5 minutes about daddy hunger are over. Life filled up also means less complaining.

- Whatever was a deficiency has turned into a sufficiency (see 2 Corinthians 12:9 NASB). We are sufficient to carry out God's will for our lives. We are equipped and not lacking the tools we need. Fullness suggests that after digestion, nutrients will be assigned to every cell, organ, and system in the body so the body can function at its best. Our minds, hearts, spirits, and relationships are more sufficient than they were during the empty seasons.

- We have energy to be the women we were created to be. It really is devastating when you know who you were created to be, but you don't have the energy to be that person. We always knew we were called for a great purpose, but daddy hunger had us lethargic, lackluster, and even lazy. Fullness has left us energized, galvanized, and revitalized.

You have supped with Abba and had your fill of Living Bread and Life-Giving Water. You might have even set up your next dinner date with Him, but maybe you'd like some more tools for living out some of His divine wisdom that we are sure He shared during dinner. Next, we will equip you with some daily practices for maintaining your healing.

Tish Granville and Lanelle Jackson

CHAPTER 9

THE INNER WORK

"The wound is how the light gets in." –Rumi

Your wounds may feel like a nuisance to you. They remind you of the hurts and harm you have survived. They take you back to the darkness. You may look at these places of wounding with shame, anger, criticism, disdain, and perhaps even fear. But your wounds are also portals of light, grace, compassion, and goodness. To move toward wholeness, you need to move toward the wounds with kindness, just as Jesus does. The following pages will teach you how to do the inner work of healing your wounds from a compassionate and gentle posture.

HEALING THE PSYCHOLOGICAL WOUNDS

Growing up without a key attachment figure in your life can leave some significant psychological wounds and even lead to serious mental health conditions and dysregulation of the mind. We cannot even begin to convey the damage that can be done by ruptured relationships. Sometimes the damage is miniscule and sometimes its mega. Our training, education and practice in clinical counseling has provided us with so much exposure to the connection between wounded minds and wounded relationships. In counseling, we rely on the Diagnostic and Statistical Manual for Mental Disorders (DSM) to diagnose and understand all existing mental and emotional disorders. Something interesting we have found is that many of the tens of diagnoses have a symptom that impacts relationships. But even more interesting is that many of the clients we have treated report that their symptoms are because of a relationship rupture or traumatic wound that occurred somewhere in their timeline, oftentimes in the parent-child system. Relationships are powerful and children fortunate enough to grow up with a secure attachment tend to enjoy more satisfying and stable relationships later in life[1] and have a decreased risk of developing mental disorders later in life. Healthy fathering and mothering are important for secure attachments.

We want to be mindful here though, especially for those who battle stigmas with mental health—fatherlessness is not a predictor that you will develop a mental health disorder. We want to establish an understanding however that fatherlessness can be a psychological wound that exists on the trauma spectrum. Depression, anxiety, and even trauma-like symptoms are not uncommon in adults who grew up in fatherless homes. In children, ADHD, conduct disorders, and oppositional-defiant disorders in addition to mood and anxiety disorders are not uncommon in fatherless homes. In most severe statistics, suicidal adolescents often come from fatherless homes. If you grew up without a father you are not just a survivor, but very likely a *trauma* survivor!

We have gone through a lot of psychological healing ourselves and we want to pass along to you some gentle, practical, and impactful resources to help you heal your psychological wound. "Resources" is a way of saying coping tools. We recommend you have both internal and external resources. Internal resources are more non-tangible like imagination, courage, joy, strength, safety, or freedom. External resources are more tangible tools like people, places, things, and activities that you can enlist into your life that are often the mode to obtaining the internal resources. For example, you can experience peace (an internal resource) by listening to music (an external resource). You can gain more security (an internal resource) by hugging a friend (an external resource). We also recommend decreasing reliance on the use of survival resources.

Survival resources are coping measures you have relied on to get through distress or stress that are not necessarily healthy and were most useful during the time of crisis or adverse life events. Once the adverse event is over, the survival resource becomes outdated. Survival resources have expiration dates on them. An example of a survival resource is "shutting down." Sometimes we shut down with people because they are abusive or damaging to us in some way and we must protect ourselves, but after we have gained freedom from the person, we still shut down, even with healthy people. The "shutting down" resource, in this case, no longer serves us; it complicates relationships. We don't need it anymore.

Look at some of the survival resources we have used that are no longer helpful:

- Shutting Down

- Silencing ourselves

- Rage

- Sleep

- Daydreaming

- Fawning/People-pleasing/Submission

We have provided for you a mix of internal and external resources to continue your healing from your daddy hunger.

Safe Place

This is an internal resource. It requires using your imagination and it does not require anything but your mind. The mind is a very powerful tool. You can imagine negatively charged or positively charged images, thoughts, or scenarios. Knowing that you have a choice in what you entertain in your mind, why not entertain healthier things? Safe place is a suitable choice. Safe place is a scene that you create in your mind of a real or imagined place that gives you the internal resource of safety and peace. When you think of this place you feel free from the feelings of anxiety, stress, and threat. Some common feelings that adults who grew up in broken homes and homes without fathers may feel are vulnerability, insecurity, anxiety, and fear. These feelings often surface during current relationship interactions and conflict. Safe place can be a helpful resource when you need alleviation within your mind. But below we have the basic steps for using this resource:

1. Find a place quiet place to sit

2. Take a few deep breaths to deepen the feeling of relaxation

3. Draw your mind inward

4. Imagine a place where you feel safe and calm; real or imagined (i.e., a beach, cabin, park, wrapped up in a blanket etc.)

5. Bring this place to mind and bring as many details into your scene as you can (i.e., colors, smells, sounds, etc.)

6. Imagine yourself there taking in all the details

7. Allow yourself to feel peaceful, calm, and safe

8. Stay in this exercise until you feel relatively balanced then resume your day

You can do this as often as you need to. Avoid judging this process and its ok if you get distracted. If you think it's silly to use this kind of imagery, we challenge you to consider the fact that you imagine things all day long. Some things that we imagine are awful and we would be embarrassed if people could see our imaginations. If you don't choose the right things to imagine, your mind will be open to very unhealthy things. God is pleased when we discipline our minds and think on very lovely things.

Journaling

To journal is to write, log, or track your personal and emotional experiences. It is a written way to chart how various experiences impact you. The goal of writing is to relieve the pressure off your heart and mind because you are transferring it all to the paper. It's a good way to keep from looping and circling over the same thoughts, feelings, and memories. Sometimes we don't know what is going on inside of us because our thoughts become tangled up like a ball of yarn, so getting it down on paper helps to untangle one string at a time. There are no rules to journaling. You can write one word or one thousand words; neatly or illegibly; once a day, once a week or once every blue moon; you can write grammatically correct or misspell every word. No rules.

We would say writing is the gateway to self-discovery for many people. To begin the healing of your psychological wound, it can be very useful to grab a pen and pad and begin the adventure of getting to know "you" and familiarizing yourself with your own hunger for dad.

Some good journal prompts are:

- I first realized I was hungry for daddy when...

- I know I'm hungry for daddy when...

- What makes me angry is...

- What makes me sad is...

- I needed my daddy when...

- I accept...

- Today I acted out my daddy hunger when...

- Today I learned that...

Meditation

To meditate is to simply concentrate on something intentionally. Do not be afraid of this word. Get rid of any previous misconceptions you have of what meditation is. In fact, don't even Google the word. You already know how to do it technically. We meditate on our fears, we meditate on our problems, we meditate on our enemies and who doesn't like us, we meditate on how to make more money—we meditate on all kinds of things already—we just don't regularly practice meditating on things that center and heal us.

We want you to consider how meditation can help to heal your psychological wounds related to your own daddy hunger.

Here is a simple guide to get you started:

Find a quiet place to sit where you will be uninterrupted. Take a few deep breaths to deepen your sense of relaxation and calmness. Recall a word, phrase, affirmation, scripture or even a scene that brings you peace. Hold the word(s) or scene in your mind while gently breathing and allow yourself to internalize it's healing power. Don't be put off by distractions, they will happen and it's ok. Just gently bring your mind back to your chosen thought. Do this for 1-10 minutes a day to begin to experience a healed mind.

Add some aromatherapy to deepen the experience. Diffusers are sold in various department stores along with basic essential oils. Go for a calming scent like lavender, lemongrass or "add your favorite scent" _____.

Deep Breathing

Your breath is your constant companion, and it is always with you, so why not use it to your advantage? Breathing is a great way to heal the mind, body and spirit and help to regulate our mood, restore our bodies, and uplift our spirits. Your breath is the reason you are alive and deep breathing sends a powerful message to your mind that even in your pain, stress, and emptiness, you are "still alive." Daddy hunger has a way of taking our breath away and/or accelerating our breath. Sometimes wounds make it hard to breathe and you just feel lifeless. Then sometimes you are in such states of worry and anxiety that your heart feels like it will pound its way out of your chest. Both extremes beg for a deep breath.

To improve your psychological health, you're going to have to breathe more intentionally. Your wound needs ventilation—a deep inhale and exhale!

Inhale acceptance-Exhale rejection
Inhale worth-Exhale worthlessness
Inhale lovability-Exhale unwantedness

Empty Chair

You learned earlier in the book about how unspoken words are swallowed, digested, and cause disruption in the heart and mind. Fatherlessness comes with a build up of words, thoughts, feelings, and all sorts of expressions that tend to get stuffed inside. Many of these stuffed words are intended to be spoken to dad—only dad is nowhere around. So, what does one do with these words? Empty chair is a healing exercise in which a speaker talks to an empty chair to get all the stuffed words, thoughts, and feelings out. The empty chair represents the person that needs to hear the words.

In our case, our father whoever he is—wherever he is—would be the person in our empty chair. We would compose our thoughts either in our heart or by first writing them down and then set up our own chair facing the empty chair that represents dad, and we would release whatever it is we want or need to say.

Now this is not a two-way conversation! It is one-way, unless you want to modify the exercise and switch seats, switch roles and respond back to your own expression from the missing person's point of view. But one-way can be very healing alone. It is the release of pent-up feelings and words that brings the unburdening. The only outcome you are expecting is to no longer feel you must carry unspoken communications within. Another modification is to sit a picture of dad on the chair opposite you if you have one and talk to the photo.

This exercise can be very powerful and evoke heavy emotions. Just imagine all the things you'd like to say to your dad, but you don't have the courage, the opportunity, the dad to say them to—you can say all these things with empty chair. Do this as often as you need to to "say what you need to say" to dad.

Affirmation

Healing words heal the mind. And you have the power to say the right words to yourself to fuse together the brokenness in your mind and heart. Affirmations are the healing words that you need to counter every negative, painful, distorted, disruptive, and disturbing word you've either said to yourself or that was said to you. You can also refer to affirmations as your "self-talk."

Affirmations can be administered verbally or through writing. Talk to yourself in the mirror, while you're in your car, in the shower, while cooking dinner, before getting out of bed in the morning or before you close your eyes at night. Affirm yourself often—with what though? — with the truth! Affirmations are statements that build you up, encourage you, validate you, compliment you, prepare you, and support you. They don't always reflect how you feel, and they don't always accurately reflect your current situation—but they teach and train you to look beyond how you feel and how things look in life.

Fatherlessness often equals a lack of affirmation as we've talked about in the book. So don't be surprised if you are in a deficit when it comes to hearing nice things about yourself or facing life's challenges with a positive attitude. Now is your time to fill your own cup with truths until your cup overflows. Give unto thyself! Speak unto thyself!

Most affirmations start with "I, I am_____, I can_____." If they don't start with "I", they most likely will have a "Me" in the statement somewhere.

We want you to feel affirmed as a survivor of daddy hunger so we have some targeted affirmations just for you in Appendix D.

Counseling

We would be remiss to not mention this as a healing tool for the psychological wounds you may have suffered from. Talking to someone who is licensed and trained in helping individuals overcome family of origin wounds, relational trauma, and childhood disturbances is invaluable. We are both counselors ourselves and we have and still receive our own counseling. Our respective counselors have been able to walk us through elements of healing we could not get to on our own even with our extensive training and knowledge. It's nice to just sit and have someone care about you and pour into you for an hour. It's the most refreshing experience to have someone ask you the right question, at the right time to help you see your pain from an angle you never approached before. It's so uplifting to have someone validate you and normalize you when you feel anything but normal because of what you've gone through. It's so supportive to have someone call out your blind spots, your patterns, your cycles, and toxic emotions and have hope for you that you can be free from them. It's also nice to have accountability to "do the work" required to overcome daddy pain. Sometimes you may find yourself retreating to unhealthy behavior because you don't have someone holding you accountable. And sometimes you may find that you're just not doing enough of the right things, and you need gentle reminders. Counseling can help with that.

When you search for a counselor, look at biographies and look for counselors who specialize or have experience in trauma, attachment disorders, relationships, family of origin issues, and grief. If you can find a Christian counselor, that is a bonus.

Self-Care/Self- Love

In recent years, self-care and self-love have become popularized and borderline clichéd recommendations. We have an idea why—It's because they are both proven to help with any ailment, stressor, illness, or trauma as well as aid in prevention from the like. Self-love is simply doing things to show kindness to yourself while self-care is doing things to maintain your overall well-being. Two different terms, but they both have the same idea in mind, which is to hold yourself in high regard and give yourself the attention you deserve.

We understand that sometimes self-love and self-care are difficult to practice if these things have not been taught to us or life challenges have derailed us from practicing them. Not to mention, we get our first lessons in self-care from the way that we are cared for.[1] If we lack the care we need from a primary caregiver, we may struggle later in life to care for ourselves or love ourselves.

Regardless of where you are in your self-care/self-love journey, it is never too late to embrace a new practice. Start small but wake up every day and decide that you will do something for yourself that is kind, thoughtful, intentional, healthy, rewarding, affirming, or beneficial.

HEALING THE RELATIONAL/SOCIAL WOUNDS

Having daddy hunger has a definite way of impacting the way you relate to others, treat others, respond to others, communicate with others, and interact with others. You could become withdrawn, overly attached, hostile, distrustful, heart-hardened, stone-cold, too trusting, or love hungry. You could develop poor boundaries or become too rigid with your boundaries and put walls up. You could draw people in or chase them away. You could become a social butterfly or a recluse. The possibilities are endless.

The concern is that most women with daddy hunger issues go to extremes. Really opened or really closed. Really softened or really hardened. Any extreme can be relationally dangerous and unhealthy. We can admit that we related and socialized in unhealthy ways during certain periods of our lives. When we were school-aged, we were a lot more withdrawn in social situations, but would go to extremes of drawing intensely to others and becoming socially clingy.

We are not judging who we were or what we did at that time, but there is a strong correlation between father absenteeism and relatability. Here are some practical solutions to build or enhance your relationships.

Resolve or Dissolve

This one may be a tough one, but it is necessary. Not all broken relationships are meant to be fixed, but all great relationships should be maintained and nurtured. Some people, God has removed from your life because they were not healthy for you, but there are some important relationships that are beneficial to you. Only you can look introspectively at your life and determine what relationships need resolved and which ones need to be dissolved. This may take some time to do but go through all the relationships you have with others and make mental notes. Are there relationships you are interested in enhancing, maintaining, or ending? You don't have to go person by person and start calling people and telling them where they stand with you, but it is important to identify where you want to be with others. We believe that the most important step is to delete unhealthy, harmful, dangerous, hostile, volatile, or roller-coaster relationships in your life. For you to heal from your daddy hunger, you certainly don't need people around you that further cause you emotional and psychological distress. You don't want to continue adding salt to old wounds by letting yourself be infected by negatively impactful relationships.

We often tell our clients to use the block feature on their phones wisely. Many of our teens and adults block people based off a mood, just to go and unblock them later. We do not encourage this. If you are deciding to block someone, this should be a permanent solution to toxicity in the relationship. This should not be used as a threat or as a game.

Build Compassionate yet Courageous Boundaries

We believe that boundaries are important in building and maintaining healthy relationships. Boundaries in relationships keep us safe.

Boundaries are not to aid us in pushing others away or cutting people off. Boundaries, if used correctly, can help bring people closer to us.

So, what are boundaries? According to Cook and Miller (2018), boundaries are the borders or limits of who you are and what you do, and what behaviors you will and will not accept.[2] To have optimal functioning in relationships or just within yourself, boundaries are necessary.

Boundaries require compassion for self and courage to speak your truth regarding your needs. They also required compassion for the other person. You are not trying to hurt the other person by asserting your limits with them.

Find a Healing Community

Healing alone can be unreasonably hard, yet so many walk alone in their journeys. We do understand that making connections requires mutual interest, you cannot force others to support you. What is within your control is remaining open to connections as they are presented to you. Look for connections with those that are supportive, wise, honest, trustworthy, and compassionate. Avoid connections with people who want to control your healing journey, over spiritualize your pain, shame you, gossip about you or want to fix you.

A healing community could also include being around individuals who can relate on some level to your story and can provide empathy.

Here are examples of individuals who could help you on your healing journey: Therapists, psychologists, psychiatrists, spiritual figures, mentors, close, but objective friends, support groups, or life coaches.

Try this simple connection mantra: "I am connected to everything and everyone that is healthy around me."

Practice Proximity Seeking

Sometimes when we experience hurt or pain from a mother or father, we go down a weary path of trying to establish healthy relationships as kids, and later, adults. We succeed in some of those relationships and fail in others. We get hurt in some of these relationships and in others, we do the hurting. We say we are done with people, then we go out of our way to get others' approval. We basically live life on a relationship teeter-totter.

Here are some simple ways you can avoid the relationship teeter-totter trend:

Attune-be mindful and stay present when you have interactions with others.

Look for ways to connect with others-don't just be a by-stander and wait for connections to come to you.

Notice when you avoid connection -practice awareness and know when you are pushing others away.

HEALING THE SPIRITUAL WOUNDS

Some of you may be wondering how someone can be spiritually wounded from growing up without a father. Well, it is possible and even likely to grow up feeling a disconnection from God or becoming confused about who God is when you experience paternal pain. Remember from Chapter 6 in the section *Parents Set the Table,* this is because earthly fathers are designed to embody the divine attributes of our Heavenly Father. Earthly fathers who are visible, connect us to God the Father, who is invisible. We then take what we experience or learn from our earthly father and develop an internal referencing system that tells us who God is, what He is like, and what He thinks about us.

The goal is for the child to develop a healthy God-concept and go through a spiritual formation process that leads them into a life-giving relationship with the Trinity. The spiritual wounding occurs when the deficits in the father-child relationship lead to doubts, disbelief, and disruptions in the Creator-creation relationship. The child believes that "God must be like my dad!" The child struggles to see God as loving, kind, present, just, and protective. What a wound!

When we were younger, we both accepted Christ and put our trust in Jesus freely. We loved Him and feared Him. We believed in Him and in many of the great attributes about Him. But there were some deficits too. We struggled, we strayed, we straddled fences regarding what we believed He thought about us and who He was as a Father to us. We knew He had the whole world in His hands, but did He have our story in His hands? He was present with us to a *degree.* He was a protector to a *degree.* He was kind to a *degree*. What degree exactly? To the same degree in which we experienced our earthly fatherlessness. This was a spiritual wound.

We bet many of you can relate to experiencing some uncertainty about your relationship with God or even going through periods where you felt His love was far from you. Experiencing relational wounds is often a precondition for survivors to begin questioning God or doubting His sovereignty. There are many scriptures that warn us not to let circumstances or people separate us from Him. But the hunger from our relationships can impair our receptivity to these admonitions.

If you feel you have gone through periods of doubting God, losing faith, or even walking completely away from God, we have some practices to get you back on track to healthy spiritual formation. Hopefully, you will understand that your earthly father had a part in causing your pain, but your heavenly Father has an even greater part in healing your pain!

Invite the Trinity into your Healing

You will need a Triune God to help recover from any trauma you have endured. God the Father, Son and Holy Spirit are instrumental in helping you integrate your pain into your life in a meaningful way. Start by sensing what each person of the Trinity (Father/Son/Spirit) means to you and what qualities each possesses. Ask each person of the Trinity to show you what you need to see about them. Then begin to sculpt conversations, questions, and prayer time around the presence of each. You will notice that acknowledging certain persons of the Trinity that you have previously ignored brings a greater quality of healing.

Connect to a Holistic and Trauma-Informed Church

We were fortunate to be a part of a large faith community and church that believed in holistic healing. The pastor of this church teaches from a socio-emotional-relational perspective, which is vital to the Gospel message. A church that offers Grief Recovery and other small groups, in addition to other traditional sacraments, is a welcomed aide in the healing process. It is important to be able to address emotional and relational wounds to become more spiritually healthy. Find a church that fits your need for Jesus and mental health. Avoid churches that demonize your depression, anxiety and trauma or places that explicitly engage in practices of spiritual abuse or practices that cause spiritual trauma.

Embody Daily Spiritual Practices

Healing from spiritual wounds requires approaching your usual spiritual disciplines from a renewed mind. Maybe you already read scripture every day and pray regularly, but you feel robotic. You are missing connection and energy. You also don't feel like your body is a part of the process. You are invited to begin bringing your body and mind into your disciplines. Experiment with new ways of praying like prayer walks, "swaying and praying", or singing your prayers. Breathe into your body when you read scripture, breathe a particular word or verse into your lungs, and try to exhale the negative spiritual trauma memories. Let worship songs soak into your nervous system where all the trauma is stored. The goal is for you to take what you've been doing for years and experience a revival deep in your viscera.

Confront Lies and Yield to Truth

We all tell ourselves certain messages based on our experiences. Oftentimes, after an unpleasant experience, an unpleasant emotion comes up, and then a thought, and then a belief. The belief therefore is directly related to the experience we had. The belief begins to hold a lot of weight and may control some of our behaviors. Simply put, we base our decisions and how we feel off a belief, a lie!

The only way to heal some of the spiritual wounds that come with fatherlessness is to explore these lies, acknowledge them, confront them, and then replace them. The best and ONLY way to replace them is to find out the truth of who God is to you and who you are to Him.

You are vital to your healing. Try not to knock or complain about what you haven't tried yet. If there is a solution that we did not list, and you want to try----try it! Be creative in your healing. Ask God (your Father) what direction you should go first. He ultimately knows what is best for you and what the best course of action to get you whole!

Of course, we hope that reading this book and using some of the resources that we provide will be the start to your healing journey. We hope that the solutions that we have provided are exactly what you need to get you un-stuck and ready to champion your emotional, relational, and spiritual health.

Tish Granville and Lanelle Jackson

CHAPTER 10

THE PATH TO YOUR PROMISE

Daddy hunger is a real problem that is plaguing our homes, communities, and the world around us. We are living witnesses that having the inner pain of a missing father is not imagined nor easily remedied. It is a devastating occurrence that has been trickling through bloodlines and generations since the biblical times. Yep! We aren't looking at a new phenomenon! We are experiencing something that God has been aware of for thousands upon thousands of years.

Let's go back briefly to the book of Genesis. Remember the story of Abraham and Sarah? Just in case you are not familiar with the story, in Genesis chapters 15-21, we see a faith-filled, yet trauma-filled story of a man, his wife, his mistress, and his two sons! Already sounds complex right? This story is chock-full of doubt, adversity, confusion, regret, wrong decisions, and disobedience. Yet we see in this story God's ability to restore, heal, bless, and uplift.

You're probably wondering, "Well, what happened?" In this compelling story, the wonderful servant Abraham and his doubtful wife Sarah were barren and without child. Sarah was very barren! They were both up in age and well past the baby-making age according to cultural expectations at that time. There was no way in Sarah's mind that she was going to give Abraham his first-born child.

While Abraham was full of faith and trusting God for a huge miracle, Sarah was full of impatience, doubt, and frustration. So, Sarah impulsively takes matters into her own hands and implores Abraham to sleep with another woman, Hagar the maidservant, to bare him a son. Well, Abraham listened to his wife and sleeps with Hagar and she becomes pregnant with Abraham's son Ishmael (See Genesis chapter 16).

After this imprudent decision, God gave Abraham a promise for a son with his wife Sarah (see Genesis 17: 1-14). She became pregnant and bore him a son (Isaac) in her old age just as God promised her. End of story, right? Everyone's happy and can go on with their lives, right? No—things became immensely complicated. Sarah was not at all happy with the outcome of having to share her husband with a mistress and a second son. So, she did what any strong-willed and insecure woman would do—she told Abraham to get Hagar and Ishmael out of here! Yep, that's right! "Send them packing and on their way because they are a distraction and there is no way I am sharing God's promise for my dear son Isaac with her and that other boy!" Well, she didn't exactly say that, but she initiated having Hagar and her son expelled from the camp.

This is where the story really becomes relatable. Abraham is left with the very difficult task of sending his mistress and first-born son packing with their bread and water bottle and out into the wilderness. They didn't have a huge supply of food, a survival kit, clothes, school money, or gas money. Just probably enough provision to last a few days.

Can you imagine how Hagar and Ishmael must have felt? Well, you don't have to wonder. Just read Genesis 21: 14-21. Hagar cried! Ishmael cried! They were devastated. They were alone, cast away, abandoned, hurt, rejected, discarded, unwanted, left to wander, and forsaken. Our hearts really go out to poor Ishmael; a young boy with no father. And let's not forget Hagar who now is a single mother. I bet you thought these sorts of things only happened present day huh? Now you can read a real story about abandonment and fatherlessness!

You have someone in the bible you can relate to and learn from. Ishmael's fatherless predicament was not his fault or desire just like you being fatherless is not your fault or desire. Fatherlessness is not something we ask for or beg God for. We do not pray while we are in the womb for God to please take our fathers away from us and leave us desolate and wandering.

But it happens! And it happens all too often! Girls and boys all over the world are left without fathers just like little Ishmael was. Some writers and scholars refer to the fatherless generation as the *Ishmael generation*. This is a generation of individuals who spend their lives wandering and living a desolate life. This is a generation with a lot of anger, hostility, pain, confusion, and rejection issues.

This is also a generation who God hears and God has great promises for! Let's look closely at Genesis 21: 15-17 (NLT).

"¹⁵ When the water was gone, she put the boy in the shade of a bush. ¹⁶ Then she went and sat down by herself about a hundred yards away. "I don't want to watch the boy die," she said, as she burst into tears. ¹⁷ But God heard the boy crying, and the angel of God called to Hagar from heaven, "Hagar, what's wrong? Do not be afraid! God has heard the boy crying as he lies there."

Wow, did you catch that? This has got to be the most phenomenal revelation regarding God hearing the cry of the fatherless. Verse 17 says God heard the lad crying! The mom was crying too, but He specifically responded with compassion and urgency to the cry of the lad.

Do you know why this verse is so useful for your healing? If you don't know why, take heart. We will paint the picture clearly for you. Right now, we want you to go back and read verse 17 again. But this time, we want you to replace "the lad" with your name. For example:

God heard (your name) crying

Now take a moment and really zone into what that means to you right now. Close your eyes and imagine the Sovereign Lord responding to every time you've cried for your earthly father. Recall all those heart-wrenching moments you sobbed in your bed, cried yourself to sleep, and cried on Father's Day. Think of when you had a life-changing moment like a birthday, graduation, or wedding and you cried because you wanted your father to be there, and he wasn't.

All your wilderness experiences where you felt alone, abandoned, and forsaken like Ishmael, God intentionally looked down on you and heard your cry. You should feel so loved and cared for just imagining that. You should also know that the same God that heard your cry then, will continue to hear your every cry. Life without a father is hard and will always pose some challenges but take heart. Every time you face a difficult or lonely moment, God will be right there to respond to you lovingly and quickly!

As we conclude, we want to show you the best part of the story of Ishmael. See verses 18-21

"¹⁸ Go to him and comfort him, for I will make a great nation from his descendants." ¹⁹ Then God opened Hagar's eyes, and she saw a well full of water. She quickly filled her water container and gave the boy a drink. ²⁰ And God was with the boy as he grew up in the wilderness. He became a skillful archer, ²¹ and he settled in the wilderness of Paran. His mother arranged for him to marry a woman from the land of Egypt."

Are you ready to celebrate? You should be because what we are about to unpack is going to reveal something life-changing for you. Here we see several things happen. First, we see God empower Hagar to ARISE. Secondly, we see God give her a command to ATTUNE to the emotional and physical needs of her son. Thirdly, we see God ANOINT Ishmael to live out his purpose.

Both Hagar and Ishmael were in states of despair and shock, leading to Hagar's isolation and dissociation from her son's condition. She reached a point where she could not attune and co-regulate with him. It was too much to watch him be in pain. Maybe she was feeling shame, guilt, anger, hopelessness and like many single moms, maybe when she saw her son, she saw her past, her mistakes, her trauma—and because of the emotional trauma, she didn't *understand the ASSIGNMENT*!

But God called her out of her state of disconnection, into a state of connection! She needed to bear witness to the fullness of her son's pain and not use defense mechanisms of denial, minimization, or dissociation. Yes, God cared about her pain, but she still had work to do! It wasn't time for her to sit down resigned. It wasn't good for her to be 100 yards away, or in the next room, or in her mom cave, or buried under the covers all day—she needed to get face-to-face with the trauma, eyeball to eyeball with her son, heart to heart with his story!

So yes, while mothers can't be fathers (chapter 7), mothers can be great mothers who co-regulate and help their children heal their father wounds. Mothers can allow God to heal their pain while they nurture and help restore their child/children in the middle of the fatherlessness wilderness experience. Mom's we know it isn't easy to be a single mom and we don't believe it is a bad thing to want your space in your grief experience. However, God was clear that he wanted Hagar to rise up out of her pain and go nurture her son because God had a promise for his life.

Despite a bad situation and being cast away from his earthly father, Ishmael was still a candidate for the blessings and promises of God. His situation was not a death sentence or a set-up for a life full of chaos and wandering. God looked on his situation and blessed him anyway. He provided for them (v.19) and He gave Ishmael a fulfilling life as an archer. But look carefully, God didn't take him or Hagar out of the wilderness. They lived there. Ishmael probably suffered from physical hunger and daddy hunger, but God provided for him. He gave him a promising life while he was there. We don't know if God sent Ishmael another father figure or a mentor, but what we do know is that God took care of him and nourished his physical and emotional body.

The same God that gave Ishmael a promising future is yet able to give you a promising future. It's so easy to fall into the belief that because you are fatherless that you are destined to lose in life and fall by the wayside. It's so easy to believe that you will never get married, never get over your hurts, never have a fulfilling career, or never be able to trust again.

We want you to believe this day and as you read the words on this page, that you are a candidate for God's promises. You are loved by God! You are heard by God! You will have a good and promising future! You will see the promises of God! You will overcome your hurts! *It is time to claim the path!*

Like Ishmael, you may still be in a wilderness experience, but that does not mean you are separated from God's promises. You can take hold and live out everything that God has for you. Don't believe the lies and don't believe you are a guaranteed statistic. There are tons of statistics that say we should all be failures, addicted, uneducated, in poverty, emotionally unstable, and criminal deviants.

We will not succumb to those stats. We stand against them in Jesus' name! We declare that we along with all of you will rise above the proclivity to live wandering miserably for the rest of our lives!

This is your official invitation to go put on your best dinner wear, clean the house, get your expensive oils (ready to pour), and gather the following: your voids, your deficits, your pangs, your story, your burdens, and your hunger—don't forget your fragmented brain and body, your hungry heart, and your starved soul—and bring this all to the *Sacred Table*. We believe there is someone Divine knocking on your door at this very moment who wants to come in and dine with you. And during this Divine Dining event, you will be unburdened of all your hunger and filled beyond what you can ask or think. All you must do is open the door! *Do you understand the assignment?*

Appendix A

20 Journaling and Art Prompts

1. What is the most painful memory I have pertaining to my father?

2. How can I stand more firmly in my identity?

3. 3 events in my life where I would have liked my father to be present.

4. What are 3 lessons I wish my dad could have/would have taught me?

5. How has my daddy hunger caused me to view God?

6. Who *saw* me during my time of hunger?

7. What do I know to be true about my journey?

8. 10 reasons why I am enough.

9. Where am I on the path to forgiveness? What does forgiveness look like for me?

10. What do I need to accept so that I may heal?

11. How do I feel about Father's Day? How do I celebrate Father's Day each year?

12. What are some ways I have coped with my daddy hunger?

13. What things have I done (positive or negative) to satisfy my cravings?

14. How am I caring for my hungry inner child?

15. How can I learn from the adversity in my life?

16. What is my definition of a good/great father?

17. Draw a picture using your non-dominant hand of your inner child

18. Draw a medal or badge that says "I survived"

19. If your life were an album, what would the playlist be?

20. 10 Things I am grateful for.

Appendix B

Scriptures for the Fatherless

Visit and look after the fatherless and widows in their distress. James 1:27 (AMP)

Never again will we say to the idols we have made, 'You are our gods.' No, in you alone do the orphans find mercy. Hosea 14:3 (NLT)

Defend the fatherless. Isaiah 1:17 (AMP)

Vindicate the weak and fatherless. Psalm 82:3 (AMP)

He ensures that orphans and widows receive justice. Deuteronomy 10:18 (NLT)

I will not leave you as orphans; I will come to you. John 14:18 (NASB)

Even if my father and my mother abandon me, the Lord will hold me close. Psalm 27:10 (NLT)

He supports the fatherless and the widow. Psalm 146:9 (NASB)

Because I rescued the poor who called, and the orphans who had no one to help them. Job 29:12

Leave your orphans behind, I will keep them alive. Jeremiah 49:11 (NASB)

You have received a spirit of adoption as sons and daughters by which we cry, "Abba! Father!" Romans 8:15 (NASB)

The victim entrusts himself to you. You alone have been the helper of the orphans. Psalm 10:14 (GW)

O Lord, you alone are my hope. I've trusted you, O Lord, from childhood. Psalm 71:5 (NLT)

Appendix C

Prayers for Daddy Hunger

Prayer for Daddy Hunger Triggers

Lord, I need your support and help right now. I am feeling the pain and burden of not having my father today. I don't want to act "out" or act "in" what I am feeling, so I need you to speak to this trigger and minister your healing to my heart and mind. Bring me to a centered place, in your name, I pray, Amen.

Prayer for Emotional Freedom

Lord, I've experienced some pain in my life and I don't like what I've allowed it to do to me. Sometimes, I feel stuck and other times I feel all over the place. I want to be free and whole in my thinking and emotions. Please help me with my emotional pain and permeate my mind with healthy thoughts and a positive outlook on life. In Jesus' name, amen.

Prayer for my Father

Lord, you know the hairs on our heads. You know everything about my dad inside and out, top to bottom. Please search my dad's heart and mind and find the places within that need your touch. If my dad is lost, please find him. If he is blind, please give him eyes to see You. If he is walking on a path that does not lead to you, please direct him. Please meet his needs according to your will and plan for his life. Protect him and keep him safe from the enemy. And if you see fit, turn his heart toward his children. In Jesus' name I pray, amen.

Prayer to Abba Father

Dear Lord, thank you for creating me and guiding my pathways throughout my life. Because of the brokenness I have experienced with my earthly father, I have struggled to see you as a father…as my father You said in your word that you will take me up when my father and mother forsake me. I have pushed you away and blamed you for my pain, but I am ready to accept you not just as God, but my father. Thank you for loving me and accepting me. From this day forward I want to receive your love and healing. I want to know you as my Abba Father. If I never have a relationship with my earthly father, I will trust you know what is best and want the very best for me as your beloved child. In Jesus' name I pray, amen.

Prayer for the Fatherless

Dear Lord, I stand in the gap today for all those who have daddy hunger. I pray that you would satisfy their hunger with good things from your heart and hand. Teach them how to persevere through their pain. Guard them from attempts to fill their voids with things and people that break your heart. Answer their questions and give them peace for all that is unknown in their journey. Supply them with father figures who will care for and support them. Some desire to be re-united with their fathers. Some will never meet their fathers. Some need to forgive their fathers. Whatever the need is, please provide for your fatherless children. And most of all, show them that You are Abba!

Prayer for Fathers

Dear Lord, you have created all of us in your image and you intentionally designed the male to be the leader of their homes and for fathers to take care of their children. Because we live in a fallen world, men everywhere have strayed away from your design. Today, I pray that you would heal men and fathers everywhere from pain and brokenness. Help them to become all that you have created them to be which is leaders, strong, spiritual, loving, whole, and present. Lord, save them and make their paths straight. Turn their hearts to you and to their children. Break the chains of hopelessness, frustration, doubt, fear, and stubbornness in your mighty name! May there be more fathers in the home than there has ever been before. May there be more fathers in the home than there are in prison, on the streets, on the run, or in the grave! Bring families back together and bring marriages back together. And it's in Your name we pray, Amen.

Prayer for Women

Dear Lord, I lift up women to You. I pray that young women would walk in integrity, wisdom, wholeness, and purpose so that when they are dating, they would do so with discernment. I pray that they would invest in relationships with men that are whole so that potential marriages would be sources of purpose and not pain that impacts generations to come. Protect your daughters from men whose hearts are hardened regarding fatherhood. Bring healing to every woman who is raising a child/children on her own and give them wisdom in how to parent, nurture, protect, and restore the woundedness their children may endure.

Prayer for Forgiveness

Dear Lord, this is hard, but help my heart to forgive. You said in Your word that You will forgive us as we forgive others. I've been hurt because of my broken relationship with my father and I find it hard to forgive him and others who have played a role in his absence or negligence. Please help me to open my heart to wave the debts of all those who have hurt me. I want to experience your promises and peace and unforgiveness keeps me trapped. I don't have to do anything extra or open myself to unnecessary hurt, but I do need to forgive so I can be free. So today, I forgive all of those who have sinned against me and everyday I will continue to forgive. Thank you God for your forgiveness and unrestricted love. Amen.

Tish Granville and Lanelle Jackson

Appendix D

Self Holds with Affirmations

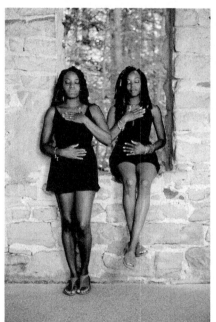

While sitting or standing, find a comfortable and relaxed posture or stance. Place one hand on your heart and the other on your abdomen (or one on your forehead and the other on your heart). Take a few deep breaths, in through your nose and out through pursed lips. As each breath goes deeper into your abdomen, allow your body to ground itself deeper into your feet or your sit bones. Continue to breathe until you feel there is a rhythm and evenness to your breath (not forced, shallow, jagged, or rigid).

As you stay in this self-hold posture, notice the sensations of touch. Feel what is happening inside of your body at the location of each hand. Notice what is happening in the space between each hand. Notice thoughts, feelings, and needs.

Once you feel settled into the self-hold, you can begin to affirm yourself.

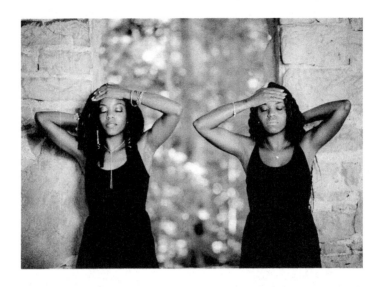

- I am worthy of love
- I am safe right now/You are safe right now
- I can ask for what I need
- I am whole/I am becoming whole
- I am enough
- It wasn't my fault
- I am not a mistake/You are not a mistake
- I am ok
- I can feel my feelings
- I have purpose/I have worth

Appendix E

Inner Child Compassion Meditation

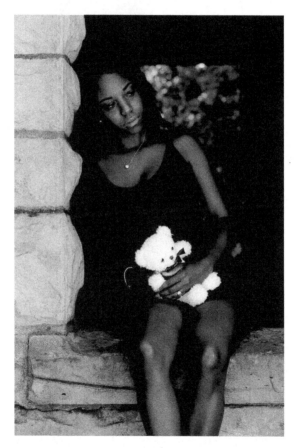

Find an object that reminds you of your inner child, like a stuffed bear, a barbie doll, a coloring book, or a picture you made. Maybe even a photo of you around a particular age.

Use the prop as an anchor to connect you to that special child that lives within you.

You can also hold/hug your inner child, with one hand positioned under your opposite arm and the other positioned over the opposite shoulder. While taking some deep breaths, speak messages of compassion to her.

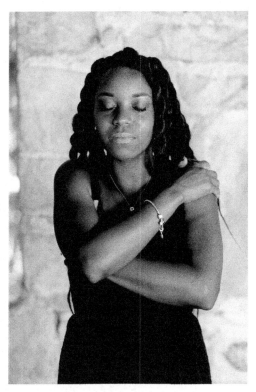

- I pray you are happy

- I pray you are healthy

- I pray you are free from your suffering

- I pray you laugh today

- I pray you have peace

- I pray you feel loved

- I pray you are whole

NOTES

Introduction Endnotes

1. https://www.worldhunger.org

2. Hunger. 2020. In Merriam-Webster.com. Retrieved August 27, 2020, from:
   http://www.merriam-webster.com/dictionary/hunger.

3. "Statistics on the Father Absent Crisis in America," Father Facts, National Fatherhood Initiative, https://www.fatherhood.org/father-absences-statistics.

Chapter 2 Endnotes

1. Brown, Brene. *Braving the Wilderness: The Quest for True Belonging and the Courage to Stand Alone.* New York: Penguin Random House, 2017.

Chapter 3 Endnotes

1. Van Der Kolk, Bessel. *The Body Keeps the Score: Brain, Mind, and Body in the Healing of Trauma.* New York: Penguin Random House, 2015.

2. Wolynn, Mark. *It Didn't Start With You: How Inherited Family Trauma Shapes Who We Are and How to End the Cycle.* New York: Penguin Random House, 2016.

3. Young, Adam. *The Place We Find Ourselves: Why Your Family of Origin Impacts Your Life More Than Anything Else.* April 16, 2018.

4. Newton, Ruth. *The Attachment Connection: Parenting a Secure and Confident Child Using the Science of Attachment Theory.* Oakland: New Harbinger Publications, 2008.

5. Porter-Gaylord, Laurel & Wolff, Ashley. *I Love My Daddy Because...*New York: Dutton Children's Books: 2004.

Chapter 4 Endnotes

1. Brewer, Judson. *The Craving Mind: From Cigarettes to Smart-Phones to Love –Why we Get Hooked & How we Can Break Bad Habits.* New Haven-London: Yale University Press, 2017.

2. McConnell, Susan. *Somatic Internal Family System Therapy: Awareness, Breath, Resonance, Movement, and Touch in Practice.* Berkley, CA: North Atlantic Books: 2020.

3. Bradshaw, John. *Home Coming: Reclaiming and Championing Your Inner Child.* United States: Bantam Books, 1990.

4. Bradshaw, John. *Home Coming: Reclaiming and Championing Your Inner Child.* United States: Bantam Books, 1990.

5. Mischke-Reeds, Manuela. *Somatic Psychotherapy Toolbox: 125 Worksheets and Exercises to Treat Trauma & Stress.* Eau Claire, WI: PESI Publishing & Media, 2018.

6. Zimberoff, Diane & Hartman, David. *Overcoming Shock: Healing the Traumatized Mind and Heart.* Far Hills, NJ: New Horizon Press. 2014.

7. Mischke-Reeds, Manuela. *Somatic Psychotherapy Toolbox: 125 Worksheets and Exercises to Treat Trauma & Stress.* Eau Claire, WI: PESI Publishing & Media, 2018.

Chapter 5 Endnotes

1. Smith, Robin. *Hungry: The Truth About Being Full.* United States: Hay House, 2013.

2. Bradshaw, John. *Home Coming: Reclaiming and Championing Your Inner Child.* United States: Bantam Books, 1990.

3. Smith, Robin. *Hungry: The Truth About Being Full.* United States: Hay House, 2013.

4. Kendall, RT. *How to Forgive Ourselves Totally*. United States. Charisma House, 2007.

5. Bradshaw, John. *Home Coming: Reclaiming and Championing Your Inner Child*. United States: Bantam Books, 1990.

6. Bradshaw, John. *Home Coming: Reclaiming and Championing Your Inner Child*. United States: Bantam Books, 1990.

Chapter 7 Endnotes

1. Johnson, Rick. *10 Things Great Dads Do: Strategies for Raising Great Kids*. Grand Rapids: Revell, 2015.

Chapter 8 Endnotes

1. Lucado, Max. *Come Thirsty: No Heart Too Dry for His Touch*. Nashville: W Publishing Group, 2004.

2. Brown, Brene. *Rising Strong: The Reckoning. The Rumble. The Revolution*. New York: Penguin Random House, 2015.

Chapter 9 Endnotes

1. Young, Adam. *The Place We Find Ourselves: Why Your Family of Origin Impacts Your Life More Than Anything Else*. April 16, 2018.

2. Cook, Alison & Miller, Kimberly. *Boundaries for Your Soul: How to Turn Your Overwhelming Thoughts and Feelings into Your Greatest Allies*. United States: Thomas Nelson, 2018.

Tish Granville and Lanelle Jackson

Tish Granville and Lanelle Jackson are available for book interviews and personal appearances. For more information contact us at info@advbooks.com, IG: @twinpowerment, Facebook: Twinpowerment

To purchase additional copies of these books, visit our bookstore at www.advbookstore.com

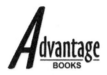

Longwood, Florida, USA
"we bring dreams to life"™
www.advbookstore.com

Made in United States
North Haven, CT
05 March 2023